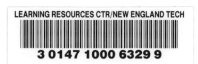

Safe and Good Use of Blood in Surgery (SANGUIS)

Use of blood products and artificial colloids in 43 European hospitals

Publication of this report has been supported by the Dissemination of Scientific and Technical Knowledge Unit, Directorate-General for Telecommunications, Information Market and Exploitation of Research, European Commission, Luxembourg

European Commission

medicine and health

Safe and Good Use of Blood in Surgery (SANGUIS)

Use of blood products and artificial colloids in 43 European hospitals

Edited by

G. Sirchia,[1] A. M. Giovanetti,[1] D. B. L. McClelland,[2] G. N. Fracchia[3]

[1] Centro Trasfusionale e d'Immunologia dei Trapianti
Ospedale Maggiore
Via Francesco Sforza 35
I-20122 Milan

[2] SES Scotland Regional Transfusion Service and
Department of Transfusion Medicine
Royal Infirmary
Lauriston Place
Edinburgh EH39HB
United Kingdom

[3] European Commission
Medical Research
DG XII-E-4
Rue de la Loi 200
B-1049 Brussels

Directorate-General
Science, Research and Development

1994   EUR 15398 EN

10-98   # 32294879

Published by the
EUROPEAN COMMISSION

Directorate-General XIII
Telecommunications, Information Market and Exploitation of Research
L-2920 LUXEMBOURG

LEGAL NOTICE

Cataloguing data can be found at the end of this publication

Luxembourg: Office for Official Publications of the European Communities, 1994
ISBN 92-826-4118-X
© ECSC-EC-EAEC, Brussels • Luxembourg, 1994
Printed in Italy

COMAC Health Services Research

This volume is the outcome of coordinated work by COMAC Health Services Research (Comité d'Action Concertée) which reports to the advisory committee on Medical and Health Research of the European Commission.

The research was carried out by the concerted action method. The European Commission pays the costs of coordination and of bringing together researchers from various countries, while the actual research is paid for and executed by each country. The aim is to accelerate joint research activities by Member States in selected fields, such as health services.

Dr Giovanni Nicola Fracchia
Secretary, COMAC Health Services Research
European Commission

Preface

This book presents the contribution and outcome of an EC concerted action (CA) on the safe and effective use of blood in surgery (Sanguis) conducted between January 1990 and June 1992 in 43 hospitals of 10 European Member States.

The objective of the CA was to assess transfusion practices in elective surgery, namely the use of red cells, whole blood, platelets, albumin and colloids in six different surgical interventions (cholecystectomy, hemicolectomy transurethral prostatectomy, coronary artery bypass graft, abdominal aorta aneurysmectomy, total hip replacement).

Other variables linked to clinical practice were also evaluated, namely the administration of drugs, laboratory data, recorded reasons which motivated transfusion, reintervention and mortality rate and length of stay in hospital.

The results of the study show a surprisingly high variability among comparable surgical teams in the different participating hospitals.

Apart from the relevance that these results have for medical practice, this study has important economic and organizational implications.

For example, for the same intervention, the preoperative stay can be 10 times longer in some hospitals than in others, and transfusion resources can be used as much as 30 times more.

In some countries, in addition, the tendency to overconsumption is evident in all participating hospitals and concerns all defined products.

The study clearly demonstrates that the variability is not linked to biological factors, but rather to the attitude of the medical profession towards blood transfusion.

This finding confirms previously published data. It also stresses the importance for all countries to try to rationalize and optimize transfusion practice.

To this purpose, consensus papers and guidelines are issued from time to time, but apparently these interventions do not succeed in significantly modifying the behaviour of the medical profession.

It is now a priority for all health systems to issue these guidelines in a more systematic way, and particularly to start collecting and analysing data in order to raise the concern of the single operator in the transfusion area, a high-cost sector where cost containment actions are becoming more and more urgent.

For this reason a copy of this book has been distributed to the 1 400 major European hospitals and centres for blood transfusion, in order to start a debate on this issue.

Paolo Fasella
Director-General, DG XII
European Commission

Sanguis Study Group

Girolamo Sirchia, MD, *Project Leader*
Centro Trasfusionale e di Immunologia dei Trapianti, Ospedale Maggiore, I—Milan

Anna Maria Giovanetti, ScD, *Project coordinator*
Centro Trasfusionale e di Immunologia dei Trapianti, Ospedale Maggiore, I—Milan

Philippe L. Baele, MD
Service d'Anesthesiologie, Cliniques Universitaires Saint Luc, B—Brussels

Rui B. Carrington da Costa, MD
Unidade de Cuidados Intensivos, Hospitais da Universidade, P—Coimbra

Nicholas Drouet, MD
Departement d'Anesthesie-Reanimation II, Centre Hospitalier Universitaire, F—Grenoble

Henk Jan ten Duis, MD
Afdeling Chirurgie, Academisch Ziekenhuis, NL—Groningen

Jan Joergensen, MD
Regional Blood Transfusion Centre, Universitetshospital, Skeiby, DK—Aarhus

Alice Maniatis, MD
Laboratory Haematology and Transfusion Medicine, University Hospital, GR—Patras

Brian McClelland, MD
SES Scotland Regional Transfusion Service and Department of Transfusion Medicine, Royal Infirmary, UK—Edinburgh

Konrad F. W. Messmer, MD
Institut für Chirurgische Forschung, Klinikum Grosshadern, D—Munich

Alvar Net Castel, MD
Servei de Medicina Intensiva, Hospital de la Santa Creu y Sant Pau, E—Barcelona

National Coordinators

Aris A. Sissouras, PhD, *Chef de File*
EC-COMAC-Health Services Research (GR)

Silvano Milani, ScD, *Biostatistician*
Centro Trasfusionale e di Immunologia dei Trapianti, Ospedale Maggiore, I—Milan

Marco Pappalettera, MD, *Biostatistician*
Centro Trasfusionale e di Immunologia dei Trapianti, Ospedale Maggiore, I—Milan

Contents

XIII

Introduction

Attitudes toward blood transfusion have changed radically in the last decade with the emergence of HIV infection, and increasing awareness of the economic crisis affecting health care in all countries. Patients are concerned about the safety of blood transfusion, payers about the costs of transfusion. Furthermore, the European Union faces major problems in meeting its own objective of self-sufficiency for blood products. [1] Against this background there is surprisingly little information about who gets transfused, why and with what effect. While studies of the use of blood in some types of surgery have been carried out, mainly in the United States, [2-5] there is no Europe-wide study of transfusion practice. Such a study is needed, to focus attention on the impact of variations in transfusion practices on clinical outcomes, the costs of care and the best use of voluntary donors' gifts. The European Commission's (EC) concerted action Sanguis was initiated to investigate transfusion practice in elective surgery in a large sample of European teaching hospitals. This report presents the principal findings of the Sanguis study.

Patients and methods

Organization

The study was performed under the contract number MR4 0237-I of the IV Medical and Health Research Programme, during a 30-month period (January 1990 to June 1992). To design and carry out the study, an international 14-member Study Group was formed with participants from the specialities of transfusion medicine, anaesthesiology, intensive care, surgery, health economics and biostatistics: 10 of the members acted as study coordinators in their respective countries.

During the preparatory phase, a standard case report form for data collection was identified; 34 junior medical doctors and four senior nurses were trained in data collection, which was accomplished between 1 October 1990 and 30 September 1991.

In each hospital, the clinicians' agreement to participate in the study was obtained by the national coordinator, as was approval of local ethics committees. Results were not fed back to the participants until completion of the study.

Hospitals

The study was performed in 158 surgical units in 43 teaching hospitals (median bed number 971) in Belgium (B), Denmark (DK), France (F), Germany (D), Great Britain (GB), Greece (GR), Italy (I), Portugal (P), Spain (E), Netherlands (NL). Two to nine teaching hospitals per country were selected by the national coordinator mainly on the basis of the willingness of clinicians to participate in providing data. This process of selection means that the contributing hospitals cannot necessarily be considered to be representative of their country.

The term 'hospital' is used throughout this report to denote one or more surgical units performing one or more of the selected operations in a given hospital. Throughout the paper, hospitals are identified by the country code followed by a letter (e.g. NL A).

Surgical procedures

Four elective surgical procedures were selected because they are frequently performed and often involve blood transfusion: right and left hemicolectomy (COLE) for colonic cancer; coronary artery bypass grafts (CABG), involving one or more vessels, arterial and/or venous grafts were distinguished; abdominal aortic aneurysmectomy (AAA), aorto-aortic, aorto-bisiliac, aorto-bifemoral grafts were distinguished; unilateral total hip replacement (THR), technical variants of procedure were not distinguished, for osteoarthritis.

Two further procedures, laparotomic cholecystectomy (CHOLE) for cholelithiasis and trans-urethral prostatectomy (TURP) for prostate adenoma, were selected as representing procedures for which blood is often ordered but rather rarely transfused.

Only first-time procedures were studied.

7

Patients

Consecutive, adult (14-90 years) patients were prospectively enrolled at the time of scheduling for surgery. Patients known to have pre-existing abnormalities of the coagulation system and those submitted to more than one surgical procedure during the episode of care were excluded. No other exclusions were made.

The size of the patient sample was set at 20 to 60 patients per surgical procedure per hospital, on the basis of a probability of 65 to 95% of observing at least one event (ordering or transfusion) occurring at a true frequency of 5% of patients operated. In hospitals where the number of operated patients over a one-year period was expected to exceed 60, the protocol limited the enrolment to the first five consecutive eligible patients in each month. Enrolment by different surgical units in the same hospital was, by protocol, proportional to each unit's share of the hospital's overall workload for that procedure.

Data

The protocol specified collection of data related to the patient, to clinical practice and to some in-hospital outcomes of surgery and transfusion.

Patient data included an identification code, age and gender, and in a sub-sample, height and weight.

Data on clinical practice identified: drugs acting on the coagulation system administered before, during and after surgery; the preoperative blood order; the type of anaesthesia used; the availability of autologous blood at surgery; the recorded blood loss; the duration of surgery; the haematocrit (Hct) or haemoglobin value on each day that a value was available (when two or more determinations were recorded in one 24-hour period, the lowest value was collected); the type and quantity of allogeneic and/or autologous blood components, albumin and artificial colloids given each day; the reasons documented in the clinical record for perioperative administration of any product.

Autologous transfusion techniques were recorded as preoperative autologous blood donation (PABD); preoperative isovolemic haemodilution (PIH); intraoperative blood salvage (IBS). The volumes of 'salvaged' blood were converted into the equivalent number of 250 mL red cell concentrates, using a published formula. [6]

Outcome variables during the hospital stay included complications of transfusion, reoperation for bleeding, and death. The length of hospital stay (LOS) was also recorded.

When an item of information could not be found by the data collector, the protocol required the entry 'not available' in the relevant section of the case report form.

The patient's clinical file was the source of information. The files of the hospital transfusion service were also searched to compare the record of requests, transfusions and transfusion complications for each patient.

Data on individual patients were, by protocol, collected during the first week after the patient's discharge from hospital.

At each hospital, or in the national coordinator's centre, data were transferred from the case report form to a specially developed application of the Paradox 3.5 database (Borland International, Scotts Valley, Ca., USA). This incorporated on-line controls for data consistency and coherence. At regular intervals, national coordinators sent copies of the local data files to the project coordinator on diskette. Before import to the central database, data were checked for completeness and compliance with coherence and consistency controls. Any inconsistent data were returned to national coordinators for review. Interim and final data analyses were performed using the Statistical Analysis System package (SAS Institute Inc., Cary, NC, USA).

Statistics

Descriptive statistics for numeric variables included the mean ± standard deviation (SD), median, the so-called hinges (i.e. 25th and 75th centile, lower and upper quartile) and range.

Confidence intervals for differences between means or percentages of characteristics of patients transfused and not transfused with red units were computed when appropriate.

The relationships between the proportion of operated patients receiving perioperative transfusion of red units (or the mean number of red units per transfused patient) and some factors (age, gender, preoperative Hct, blood loss, administration of drugs acting on the coagulation system (for THR), type of graft (for CABG and AAA), type of anaesthesia (for THR)) were evaluated within the hospital (so as to avoid the confounding effects of the above relationships due to the differences in the distribution of the variables among hospitals). Hospitals where 90% or more or 10% or less of patients receiving transfusion for a given procedure were excluded from this analysis. Continuous variables (e.g. Hct and blood loss) were recoded into three categories, using the two tertiles of their distribution as cut-off points.

Data analysis was performed by fitting general linear models, [7] including as terms: the hospital, the above factors and their first degree of interaction. Results were expressed as least squares means (± standard error, SE) based on the model, and hence adjusted for the other terms in the model.

Because there were many empty cells for some items of data when all the above factors were simultaneously considered, we were required to fit models including a reduced number of variables. Thus, the effect of age (or gender) was adjusted for hospital and gender (or age), but

9

not for the remaining factors; the effect of each further factor was adjusted for hospital, age and gender. Only in the case of preoperative Hct and blood loss, were the two factors simultaneously included in the model. In any case, the adjustment tends to remove the bias in the estimate of the effect of a factor on the occurrence of transfusion, when the other factors in the model also exert their effects. The effect of autotransfusion on overall red unit use was studied by comparing the results obtained from three groups of hospitals, formed according to an arbitrary percentage of the transfused patients who received autologous red units with or without allogeneic ones (<10%, 10 to 50%, >50%).

As a rule of thumb, differences were considered not to be due to chance when they exceeded three times the standard error.

We estimated the relative risk (RR) for a patient of being transfused in hospitals of central-northern Europe (Belgium, Denmark, France, Germany, Great Britain, Netherlands) compared with that for a patient in hospitals of the Mediterranean area (Greece, Italy, Portugal, Spain). Estimates were adjusted for age and gender, using the Mantel-Haenszel method and test-based 95% confidence interval. [8] Results were expressed as RR (95% confidence interval).

Hospitals with less than 20 patients per surgical procedure per hospital, as well as reoperated patients and patients dying during the hospital stay, were excluded from inferential data analysis, but these patients were included in the descriptive analysis.

Costs

To make a rough calculation of the costs of blood products used, we averaged values of cost or price information provided by blood transfusion services of six participating countries. The average costs per unit were: whole blood or red cell concentrate (both allogeneic and autologous) = ECU 60; recovered plasma and platelet concentrate = ECU 25. The average price of albumin was ECU 2.2/g. The price of artificial colloids, including any solution of gelatin, dextran and hydroxyethyl starch (HES), was taken as ECU 0.025/mL. Cumulative costs were expressed in ECUs per operated patient by hospital for each surgical procedure.

The costs of a preoperative request to the transfusion service for pretransfusion tests (ABO, Rh group and red cell antibody screening) was taken as ECU 10 per patient.

The Sanguis study: the background

The first step was the submission (September 1989) of a declaration of intent to the European Commission (Biomedical and Health Research Programme's call for proposal) by Prof. Girolamo Sirchia, Medical Director of the Centro Trasfusionale e di Immunologia dei Trapianti, Ospedale Maggiore Policlinico, I-Milano, on the basis of a previous experience performed at his setting. [9, 10] The Sanguis project was approved in January 1990 and the allocated financial support for the international coordination was ECU 308 000/30 months.

The scheduled timetable and phases of the study accomplishment are illustrated below:

January 1990 *	June *	October * * *	September 1991 *	June 1992 *
Set-up	Pilot phase	Data collection		Conclusion
study group design organization training course		interim analysis		final analysis dissemination of results

* indicates workshops

Set-up phase (January to June 1990)

1. The Sanguis study group was formed by the project initiator. Eleven professionals, representing different medical specialities of various EU countries, and with experience and interest in transfusion, were invited. All who were invited agreed to participate. In addition to support from the COMAC secretariat, a member of the EC COMAC advisory group participated in the study as 'chef de file'. Ten of the study group members acted as national coordinators of the project, one as project leader and one as project coordinator. In addition, two biostatisticians were included.
The study group was charged with the design and setting-up of the project, including development of the case report form, identification of the participating hospitals, selection, training and support of the data collectors, raising funds at national level, control of data collection and reliability, and assistance to the project leader.

2. Case report form. This was widely discussed during two workshops. After clarification of the project aims and definition of the type and amount of data to be collected, it was decided to use a prospective patient enrolment. The collection of data, however, was not prospective or concurrent, since it was considered that this would influence the normal clinical practices of data recording. Data were therefore collected during the week following the patient's discharge from the surgical unit. It was assumed that completed clinical records would generally be accessible to the data collectors during this period.
The study group were concerned about the quantity of data to be obtained to complete each case report form, but concluded that this unique opportunity should be used to obtain as complete a view of transfusion practice as possible.

3. Establishment of a scientific secretariat at the department of the project leader, charged with overall coordination, training of the data collectors, development of the computerized programme, data management and analysis. The secretariat comprised a full-time senior researcher, a part-time junior researcher, two part-time data managers/processors, two part-time statisticians and a part-time secretary. The development and implementation of the computerized program was challenging due to the relative complexity of the case report form and programming of the controls for coherence and consistency.

4. Training course for staff charged with data collection. The aim was to establish full understanding of definitions and conventions, to establish uniform working practices and to familiarize staff with the computerized case report form.

5. Rules for publication. The relevant paper was prepared by one of the national coordinators (Prof. K. Messmer, D) and signed by all members.

11

Pilot phase (July to September 1990)

The pilot phase, involving 1 165 patients from 23 hospitals located in seven countries, showed the feasibility of the project and adequacy of the organization, although there were problems to be solved with the computerized program. The data analysis of the pilot study was performed and results partly published. After the pilot study, it was decided that for each surgical procedure only one pathological diagnosis would be selected. Two of the initial participating hospitals (originally 45) withdrew due to difficulties with data collection.

Data collection and interim data analysis (October 1990 to September 1991)

During the year of data collection, four interim data analyses were performed and discussed during four workshops held with the national coordinators, one also with the participation of the data collectors. Approaches to the analysis and presentation of the data were extensively discussed at these workshops. After each workshop, reports were regularly sent to each national coordinator and the EC.

Final data analysis

8 126 case report forms were received by the secretariat in 120 separate mailings. Overall, eight (0.1%) case report forms were not accepted because part of the information was lacking, and 1 032 (13%) were returned for review by the national coordinator. Before data analysis, 580 (7%) of 8 118 case report forms still showed one or more incongruous pieces of information, corresponding to 0.7% (580/82 000) of the total number of data fields. Examples of these were:

  (i) no specification (e.g. blood units were requested but the number was not documented)
 (ii) outlier (e.g. LOS was longer than the pre-fixed term of 60 days)
(iii) blank (i.e. no entry)[1]
 (iv) incoherence (e.g. date of hospital admission > than that of surgery)[1]
  (v) error (e.g. digit of a nonsense code)[1]

Uncorrected erroneous, incoherent and blank fields were excluded from analysis, while outliers and unspecified fields were included as such.

Nine hundred and twenty-three (11%) case report forms relating to the procedure of laparoscopic cholecystectomy, subtotal colectomy, abdomino-perineal rectal amputation and open prostatectomy were excluded from analysis because hospitals enrolling 20 or more patients were only four, two, two, and two in number respectively, while the remaining 7 195 (89%) case report forms referring to laparotomic cholecystectomy, transurethral resection of the prostate, right and left hemicolectomy, coronary artery bypass graft, abdominal aorta aneurysmectomy and total hip replacement were analysed. These represented 76.4% of the planned 60 patients per surgical procedure per hospital in the year of data collection. In three hospitals the difference between planned and collected data was due to difficulties in obtaining data, while in the remaining 31 hospitals it was due to either a change in the surgical activity performed or to a lower level of surgical activity than had been expected.

---

[1] Observed with the use of a preliminary version of the program.

The proportion of hospitals enrolling less than 20 patients varied from 9% (CABG) to 35% (AAA), according to the surgical procedure. Furthermore, 4% of patients were from 18 hospitals reporting less than 20 patients for one or more surgical procedures.

Since not all hospitals carried out all the surgical procedures to be studied, national coordinators had to select hospitals that together could provide the planned range and number of cases.

Sanguis, being a multicentre exercise in the collection, analysis and dissemination of a very complete set of data, provided a number of substantial challenges in the following aspects:

  (i) methodology:
       type of study,
       sample size,
       patient inclusion and exclusion criteria,
       timing,
       type and amount of data,
       data collection:
       computerization,
       monitoring (interim analysis),
       data analysis;
 (ii) communication;
(iii) coordination;
(iv) support.

Advantages of the study's design included the following:

  (i) large patient sample and broad origin of the data;
 (ii) harmonization of methodology;
(iii) cooperation, both national and international and among a wide range of disciplines.

Results

Results are given in two parts: the first part includes an overview and the second presents the detailed findings for each surgical procedure

Part I
Overview

Patients

In all 7 195 case report forms were available for analysis: 64% from 23 hospitals in six countries of central-northern Europe, and 36% from 20 hospitals in four countries of the Mediterranean area. Table 0.1 reports the number of patients according to surgical procedure and hospital.

Table 0.1. Number of patients enrolled for each surgical procedure in each hospital

Country	Hospital code	CHOLE	COLE	TURP	CABG	AAA	THR	Number by hospital	Number by country
Belgium	BA	11	59	54	75	48	77	324	
	BB	13	59	12	78	61	54	277	
	BC	9	50	67	67	27	58	278	879
Germany	DA	35	31	35	71	26	16	214	
	DB	61	32	7	34	8	40	182	396
Denmark	DKA	38	46	59	60	41	63	307	
	DKB	25	52	62			63	202	
	DKC	60	12	60	62	57	62	313	822
Spain	EA	32	50	1	11	3	4	101	
	EB	58	14	60			10	142	
	EC	59	54	59	58	13	58	301	
	ED	33	11		1	9	12	66	610
France	FA		36				41	77	
	FB	45	14	104	63	49		275	
	FC	57	45	55	30	32	59	278	
	FD	64	57					121	751
United Kingdom	GBA				72	55		127	
	GBB			35				35	
	GBC						72	72	
	GBD	48	42	30				120	
	GBE	55	54	66		8		183	
	GBF	92		53	72	1	64	282	
	GBG	72	30	73	72			247	
	GBH						72	72	
	GBI						68	68	1 206
Greece	GRA						80	80	
	GRB	84						84	
	GRC		27					27 [1]	
	GRD						92	92	
	GRE					50		50	
	GRF						62	62	395
Italy	IA	101	36	16		58		211	
	IB						108	108	
	IC						71	71	
	ID	95	44	74	84	49	64	410 [2]	
	IE	31	8	11			10	60	
	IG				26	41	55	122	
	IH				55	13	13	81	
	IL	59	21	62			38	180	1 243 [2]
Netherlands	NLA	44	36	39	62	22	63	266	
	NLB	68	39	50		21	76	254	520
Portugal	PA	112	22	13	70			217	
	PB	43	14	33	43	1	22	156	373 [1]
10	43	1 504	995	1 190	1 166	693	1 647	7 195	

CHOLE = laparotomic cholecystectomy
COLE = right and left hemicolectomy
TURP = transurethral prostatectomy
[1] minimum value.

CABG = coronary artery bypass graft
AAA = abdominal aorta aneurysmectomy
THR = total hip replacement
[2] maximum value.

19

Figure 0.1 shows the number of patients enrolled in each hospital, expressed as a proportion of the number of enrolments in the hospital that provided the largest number of patients.

Of the 7 195 patients, 468 (6%) were included in the descriptive statistics but were excluded from inferential analysis either because they were from hospitals that enrolled less than 20 patients for one or more surgical procedures (4%), or because they underwent a reintervention (1%) or died (1%) during the hospital stay.

A summary of patient characteristics and data related to surgery is shown in Table 0.2 for each surgical procedure. This illustrates the wide differences that exist among the patients from the study hospitals for each variable within all the categories of surgical procedure.

Table 0.2. Characteristics of patients and some variables related to surgery

	Chole-cystectomy (CHOLE)	Right and left hemicolectomy (COLE)	Transurethral prostate resection (TURP)	Coronary artery bypass graft (CABG)	Abdominal aorta aneurysm-ectomy (AAA)	Total hip replace-ment (THR)
Number of patients	1 504	995	1 190	1 166	693	1 647
age, median year number	58 (47-71)	68 (63-75)	71 (59-75)	62 (58-71)	69 (66-71)	66 (58-77)
men (% patients)	32 (11-46)	50 (25-86)	100	83 (64-100)	90 (0-100)	35 (18-61)
Preoperative length of hospital stay, median day number	2 (1-12)	4 (2-15)	2 (1-14)	3 (1-11)	4 (1-17)	3 (1-13)
Preoperative haematocrit, median value, %	40 (37-42)	38 (34-41)	43 (40-46)	42 (39-45)	42 (38-47)	40 (36-43)
Regional or combined anaesthesia (% patients)	3 (0-23)	12 (0-87)	68 (0-100)	0.5 (0-8)	29 (0-96)	31 (0-100)
Anticoagulant drug administration[1] (% patients)	25 (0-91)	28 (0-100)	20 (0-98)	89 (3-100)	59 (2-100)	51 (0-100)
Anticoagulant and haemostatic drug administration[1] (% patients)	0.1 (0-9)	0.1 (0-2)	0.0 (0-2)	21 (0-100)	0.1 (0-6)	0.1 (0-2)
Graft (% patients)						
mammary artery				13 (0-81)		
both mammary and saphenous, or other venous graft				60 (0-100)		
saphenous vein				27 (0-79)		
aorto-bifemoral					26 (0-55)	
aorto-bi-iliac					35 (5-67)	
aorto aortic termino-terminal					39 (0-87)	
Duration of surgery, median minute number[2]	90 (45-140)	150 (90-185)	60 (40-190)	230 (72-360)	180 (160-320)	110 (60-180)
Blood loss volumes, median litre number[2]	0.2 (0.0-0.2)	0.4 (0.1-0.8)	0.5 (0.4-0.5)	0.6 (0.3-0.9)	1.3 (0.5-2.2)	0.6 (0.4-1.0)

Note: In parentheses, the lowest-highest value observed among hospitals.
[1] From admission to surgery.
[2] When recorded in 50% or more of operated patients.

Transfusion data

Of the 7 195 patients, 2 441 (34%) were transfused with 11 474 units of allogeneic blood components, 500 (7%) with 1 434 units of autologous blood components, 640 (9%) with both

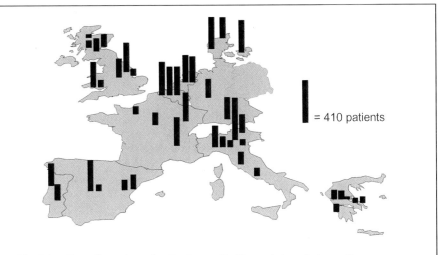

Fig 0.1. - Overall number of patients enrolled in each hospital over the one-year period, regardless of the type of surgical procedure, expressed as proportion of the number of enrolments in the hospital providing the largest number of patients

1 597 autologous and 3 178 allogeneic units. In 84 patients (1%) the record of the number and type of blood components was incomplete. 1 566 patients (22%) received 123 693 g of albumin and 2 517 patients (35%) 3 022 L of artificial colloids.

Table 0.3 shows, by surgical procedure, the percentage of operated patients who were transfused with each product and the quantity of each product given per recipient. Again, wide differences among hospitals are evident. The table also shows that autologous blood was predominantly used in CABG, AAA and THR, and plasma and albumin in CABG and AAA.

Table 0.3. Transfusion data

	Cholecystec-tomy (CHOLE)	Right and left hemicolectomy (COLE)	Transurethral prostate resection (TURP)	Coronary artery bypass graft (CABG)	Abdominal aorta aneurysmectomy (AAA)	Total hip replacement (THR)
Red units [1]						
percentage of operated patients transfused with red units						
total	3.8 (0-8)	40.9 (0-79)	16.5 (0-46)	87.7 (17-100)	82.7 (64-100)	80.8 (29-100)
allogeneic	3.7 (0-8)	38.5 (0-79)	15.4 (0-34)	37.6 (0-96)	53.7 (7-100)	56.8 (0-100)
autologous	0.1 (0-3)	1.9 (0-25)	0.8 (0-15)	14.6 (0-100)	13.0 (0-67)	15.6 (0-80)
allogeneic and autologous		0.5 (0-12)	0.3 (0-8)	35.5 (0-91)	16.0 (0-58)	8.4 (0-50)
median number of units per patient transfused with red units						
total	2 (−)	2 (1-4)	2 (1-3)	4 (1-5)	3 (2-7)	3 (2-5)
allogeneic	2 (−)	2 (2-4)	2 (2-3)	3 (2-5)	3 (2-5)	3 (2-4)
autologous	—	2 (2-2)	1 (1-2)	2 (1-3)	2 (1-3)	2 (2-3)
allogeneic and autologous	—	—	—	5 (3-6)	6 (4-9)	4 (3-6)
Plasma						
percentage of operated patients transfused with plasma	1 (0-8)	10 (0-57)	1 (0-15)	39 (0-100)	26 (0-100)	6 (0-95)
median number of units per transfused patient	2 (−)	4 (2-6)	2 (−)	4 (1-10)	4 (1-8)	2 (2-2)
Platelets						
percentage of operated patients transfused with platelet concentrates	0.1 (0-1)	0.2 (0-4)	0.0 (0-2)	7.7 (0-38)	2.6 (0-12)	0.2 (0-2)
median number of units per transfused patient	—	—	—	6 (4-8)	5 (−)	—
Albumin						
percentage of operated patients receiving albumin	3 (0-67)	32 (0-98)	3 (0-19)	54 (0-100)	46 (0-100)	13 (0-76)
median number of grams per administered patient	21 (16-21)	62 (11-126)	21 (21-21)	64 (21-226)	61 (26-122)	26 (9-41)
Artificial colloids						
percentage of operated patients receiving colloids	8 (0-59)	36 (0-94)	20 (0-89)	48 (0-100)	64 (0-100)	49 (0-98)
median volume per administered patient, L	0.5 (0.5-0.5)	0.5 (0.5-1.0)	0.5 (0.5-0.5)	1.0 (0.5-4.0)	1.0 (0.5-1.9)	0.5 (0.5-2.5)

Notes: (i) Blank cells indicate 0; (ii) in parentheses, the lowest-highest value observed among hospitals; (iii) — = quantities not calculated (number of transfused patients < 6).

[1] Red units = units of whole blood or red blood cell concentrates.

Type of products

Regardless of the surgical procedure, blood components were used together with albumin and artificial colloids in 27 of 43 hospitals (63%), nearly three quarters of which were located in central-northern Europe (Figure 0.2). Figure 0.2 also shows hospitals where the use of given products varied in accordance with the surgical procedure, and hospitals where the same products were used irrespective of surgical procedure.

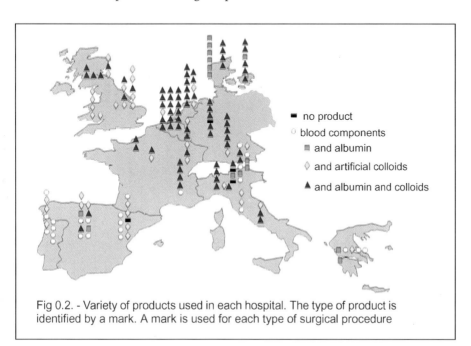

Fig 0.2. - Variety of products used in each hospital. The type of product is identified by a mark. A mark is used for each type of surgical procedure

1.0. *Red units*

For each procedure there was an enormous variability in the percentage of patients transfused among hospitals, even those within a single country. In hospitals of central-northern Europe, the percentage of patients transfused with red units was similar to that observed in those of the Mediterranean area for CABG, AAA, and CHOLE, while it was significantly lower for TURP (RR = 0.6 (0.5 to 0.8)), COLE (RR = 0.8 (0.6 to 0.9)) and THR (RR = 0.4 (0.3 to 0.6)).

A median of two red units was transfused in nearly three quarters of the hospitals performing COLE and TURP, and in half of those performing THR. Even larger variations were seen among the hospitals performing CABG and AAA.

1.1. *Autologous red units*

Autotransfusion was used by the large majority of the hospitals located in the Mediterranean area but only by a half or less (according to procedure) of the hospitals of central-northern Europe (Figure 0.3). In the latter area, moreover, the percentage of autotransfused patients was significantly lower in CABG (RR = 0.5 (0.5 to 0.6)), in AAA (RR = 0.4 (0.3 to 0.5)) and in THR (RR = 0.0 (0.0 to 0.1)).

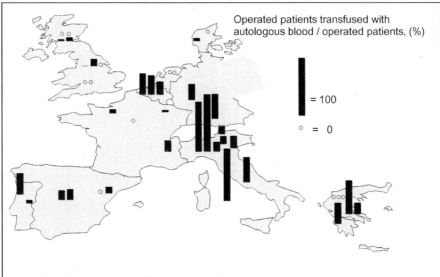

Operated patients transfused with
autologous blood / operated patients, (%)

= 100

° = 0

Fig 0.3. - Use of autotransfusion at each hospital, regardless of the surgical
procedure

When the various techniques of autotransfusion are considered, PABD was prevalent in THR
providing 1.5 times the units obtained from other autotransfusion techniques, whereas IBS was
prevalent in CABG and AAA (two and four times the units provided by other autotransfusion
techniques, respectively). A combination of two or three different techniques was employed in a
half to two thirds of the hospitals depending on the surgical procedure.

1.2. Whole blood

Of all allogeneic red units, 16% were transfused as whole blood. This percentage varied from
3% (TURP) to 31% (THR) according to the surgical procedure and from 0 to 100% according
to the hospital. The proportion was particularly high in some hospitals of two countries (Figure
0.4). In three of nine hospitals in Great Britain, whole blood units constituted 44 to 77% of all
the red units transfused. Similarly, in three of six Greek hospitals, 52 to 100% of all the red
units were transfused as whole blood.

2.0. Platelets

Platelets were used in 24 of the 43 hospitals (Figure 0.5). Of platelet recipients, 77% were
CABG patients (69% were in four hospitals). A further 15% of platelet recipients were AAA
patients.

3.0. Plasma

Plasma was used in 37 of the 43 hospitals (Figure 0.6). For CABG, about 50% of plasma
recipients (and units) were in four hospitals, for AAA in five, and for COLE in four.

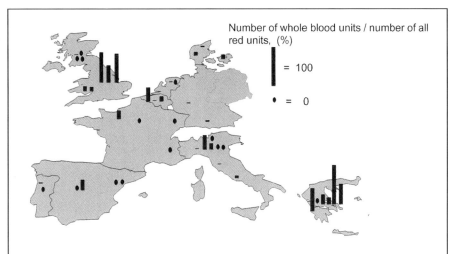

Fig 0.4. - Overall proportion of allogeneic red units used as whole blood in each hospital

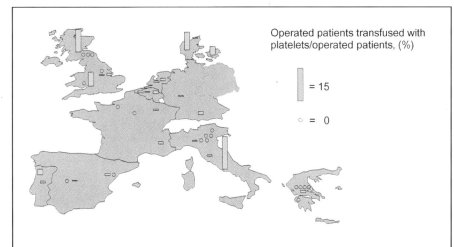

Fig 0.5. - Overall use of platelet concentrates in each hospital

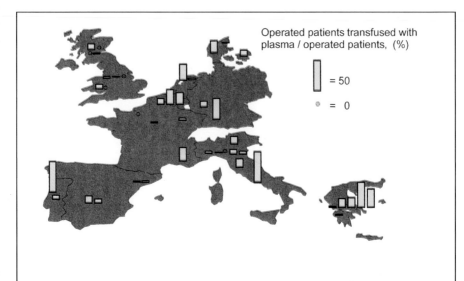

Operated patients transfused with
plasma / operated patients, (%)

= 50

= 0

Fig 0.6.- Use of of plasma at each hospital, irrespective of the surgical procedure

The percentage of patients transfused with plasma in central-northern Europe was similar to that observed in the Mediterranean area for AAA, while it was higher for CHOLE, COLE, TURP and CABG, and lower for THR.

Of plasma recipients, 92% also received red units during their hospital stay and 81% on the same day.

3.1. Type of plasma

The proportion of liquid plasma used was considerable (Figure 0.7). This component was used in eight hospitals (Figure 0.8), in seven of which it constituted 60 to 100% of all plasma units used. Plasma from apheresis was used in five hospitals and in three of them (BA, BC, IA) it accounted for 52 to 100% of the plasma units there transfused.

Lyophilized plasma was used by only three hospitals and in a total of only three patients (GRB for CHOLE, ED and BC for COLE).

4.0. Cryoprecipitate

Cryoprecipitate was used in 10 hospitals (Figure 0.9). In all 107 units were given to 10 CABG patients and 37 to eight AAA patients. Of all the units, 55% were transfused in one hospital (GBA).

5.0. Albumin

Albumin was used in 30 of the 43 hospitals (Figure 0.10). The percentage of patients given albumin in hospitals located in central-northern Europe was, according to procedure, 2 to 10 times higher than that observed in the Mediterranean area (RR ranging from 2 (2 to 3) in COLE to 10 (7 to 13) in AAA).

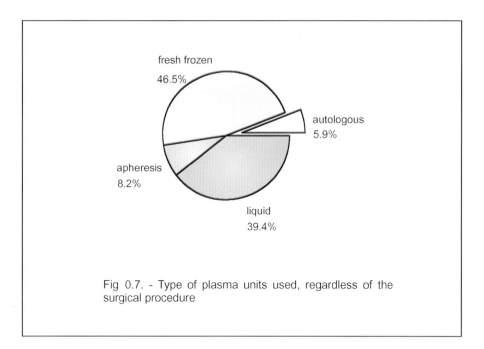

Fig 0.7. - Type of plasma units used, regardless of the surgical procedure

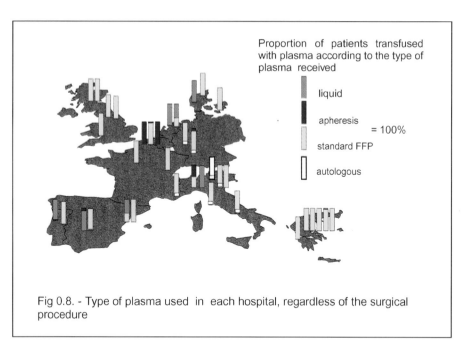

Fig 0.8. - Type of plasma used in each hospital, regardless of the surgical procedure

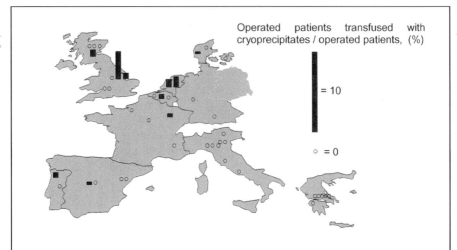

Fig 0.9. - Use of cryoprecipitates in each hospital, regardless of the surgical procedure

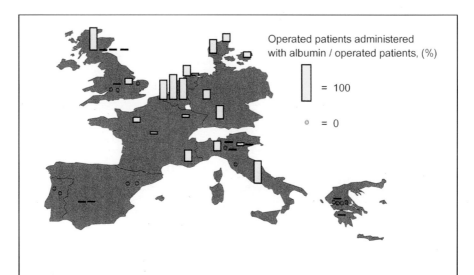

Fig 0.10. - Use of albumin at each hospital, regardless of the surgical procedure

The greatest use of albumin was observed in the three Belgian hospitals, accounting for 38% of all albumin recipients and 44% of all albumin used in the entire study. This high use was observed in nearly all surgical procedures.

6.0. *Artificial colloids*

Of the 43 hospitals, 35 used artificial colloids (Figure 0.11). Of these, 13 used mainly gelatin, four mainly dextran, two mainly hydroxylethyl starch (HES) and those remaining used two or three different artificial colloids in varying proportions.

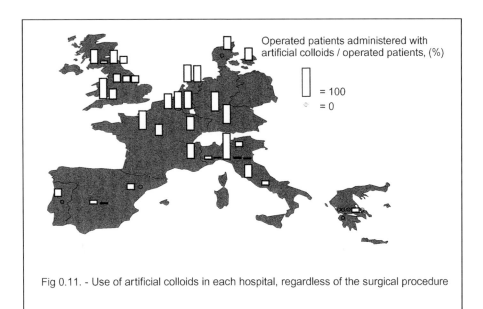

Fig 0.11. - Use of artificial colloids in each hospital, regardless of the surgical procedure

The overall percentage of recipients and volumes according to the type of colloid is displayed in Figure 0.12.

The percentage of patients receiving artificial colloids in central-northern Europe was significantly higher than in hospitals located in the Mediterranean area (RR ranging from 3 (2 to 3) in AAA to 101 (43 to 239) in CHOLE). As with albumin, the greatest use of artificial colloids was in the three Belgian hospitals, which together used 36% of the total quantity. This high use of colloids was seen in nearly all surgical procedures.

Time of transfusion

Regardless of the product, transfusions were, as expected, most frequently given during the perioperative period (Table 0.4), the lowest value being observed in COLE and the highest in CABG. For nearly all products, wide differences in the times that patients were transfused were observed among hospitals.

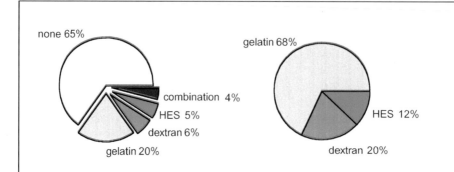

Fig 0.12. - Use of artificial colloids, irrespective of the surgical procedure. On the left: distribution of overall operated patients according to the type of artificial colloid received. On the right: proportion of the total volume of artificial colloid administered by type

Table 0.4. Distribution of transfused patients according to the time of transfusion in respect to surgery

Surgery	Time of transfusion	Red units	Percentage of transfused patients Plasma	Platelets	Albumin	Artificial colloids
CHOLE	preoperative	8.6 (0-50)	13.6 (11-100)		4.3 (0-17)	3.3 (0-20)
	perioperative	69.0 (0-100)	59.1 (0-100)		82.6 (0-100)	95.1 (0-100)
	postoperative	12.1 (0-67)	9.2 (0-100)	50 (-100)		0.8 (0-100)
	more than one time	10.3 (0-100)	18.1 (11-50)	50 (-100)	13.1 (0-100)	0.8 (0-50)
COLE	preoperative	9.8 (0-33)	1.9 (0-100)			0.6 (0-6)
	perioperative	65.6 (0-84)	76.9 (0-100)	100	69.4 (0-100)	97.5 (72-100)
	postoperative	8.8 (0-75)	9.6 (0-33)		3.2 (0-100)	0.3 (0-17)
	more than one time	15.8 (0-32)	11.6 (0-33)		27.4 (0-100)	1.6 (0-22)
TURP	preoperative	3.5 (0-50)			2.7 (0-50)	0.4 (0-5)
	perioperative	81.7 (50-100)	82.3 (0-100)	100	97.3 (50-100)	99.6 (95-100)
	postoperative	5.1 (0-25)	11.8 (0-100)			
	more than one time	9.7 (0-50)	5.9 (0-100)			
CABG	preoperative	0.2 (0-3)	0.4 (0-5)		0.5 (0-2)	0.4 (0-1)
	perioperative	92.3 (70-100)	97.1 (74-100)	95.6 (0-100)	92.6 (78-100)	97.3 (83-100)
	postoperative	0.8 (0-21)	0.7 (0-25)	1.1 (0-9)	0.2 (0-7)	0.3 (0-11)
	more than one time	6.7 (0-21)	1.8 (0-9)	3.3 (0-100)	6.7 (0-18)	2.0 (0-17)
AAA	preoperative					
	perioperative	87.8 (59-100)	94.5 (50-100)	88.9 (50-100)	90.9 (50-100)	93.4 (40-100)
	postoperative	1.9 (0-33)	2.2 (0-50)	11.1 (0-50)	0.6 (0-50)	0.4 (0-14)
	more than one time	10.3 (0-28)	3.3 (0-9)		8.5 (0-100)	6.2 (0-60)
THR	preoperative	0.4 (0-8)	2.8 (0-12)			0.4 (0-2)
	perioperative	84.4 (50-100)	89.6 (71-100)	100	95.8 (50-100)	90.6 (27-100)
	postoperative	3.0 (0-50)	2.8 (0-28)		2.3 (0-100)	
	more than one time	12.2 (0-42)	4.8 (0-17)		1.9 (0-9)	9 (0-72)

Blank cells = 0.
Perioperative = from the day of surgery to three days after (inclusive).
Postoperative = from the fourth day after surgery to discharge.

Documented reasons for perioperative transfusion

Only 23% of the clinical records of patients receiving red units contained a documented reason for transfusion. A low Hct (of 28% ± 3, mean and median, ± SD) or the presence of bleeding were the most frequently documented reasons for transfusion. In only four of the 43 hospitals was the reason for transfusion documented for 50% or more of the transfused patients (Figure 0.13). In relation to the surgical procedure, reasons for transfusion documented in the clinical records varied from 17% (CABG) to 30% (CHOLE).

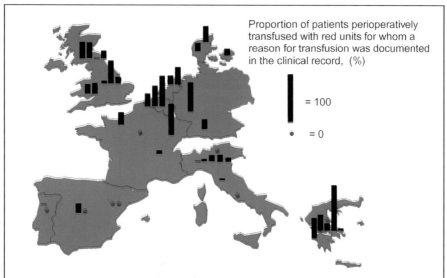

Proportion of patients perioperatively transfused with red units for whom a reason for transfusion was documented in the clinical record, (%)

= 100

• = 0

Fig 0.13. - Reasons for perioperative red unit transfusion documented in the medical record at each hospital, irrespective of the surgical procedure

The records of 26% of the patients receiving plasma contained a reason for plasma transfusion. A prothrombin time result was found in 16% of the recipients: the test result was below 60% of control in only 12% of the recipients. For 6% of plasma recipients, volume replacement was the reason given for transfusion. The presence of a documented reason to transfuse varied, according to the surgical procedure, from 7% (THR) to 38% (COLE).

A reason for platelet transfusion was documented only in CABG for 32% of the recipients and in AAA for 25%. The presence of bleeding was the indication most frequently reported. In CABG, a platelet count was recorded in 7% of platelet recipients: the values ranged from 36 to 88x10⁹/L.

A reason for the administration of albumin was recorded in 13% of the recipients and for artificial colloids in 17%. In most cases the stated indication was volume replacement. The majority of these records were from Belgian hospitals.

31

Variables associated with perioperative transfusion of red units

The effect of some variables on the probability of an operated patient being transfused is described in the sections dealing with each procedure. In summary (Figure 0.14), females, after adjustment for age, were significantly more likely to be transfused than males in both of the two procedures where this variable was evaluated. Increasing age was associated with a higher probability of patients being transfused in COLE, CABG and AAA. Furthermore, the higher the preoperative Hct value, the lower the probability of transfusion, while the higher the blood loss, the higher the probability of transfusion, even after adjustment for age and gender.

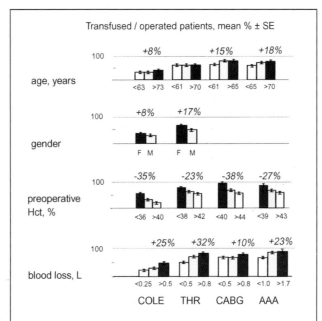

Fig 0.14. - Effect of age, gender, preoperative hematocrit value (Hct) and blood loss on the proportion of patients perioperatively transfused with red units in right and left hemicolectomy (COLE), total hip replacement (THR), coronary artery bypass graft (CABG), and abdominal aortic aneurysmectomy (AAA). On the x axis, the values of the lowest and highest class are shown for each variable. Numbers in italics indicate the difference in the proportion of patients transfused that is attributable to each factor. The effect of age (gender) was adjusted for gender (age), whereas that of preoperative Hct or of blood loss for both age and gender (COLE and THR)

The probability of a patient being transfused in hospitals that frequently use autotransfusion was significantly higher than in those with a low use of autotransfusion (86% ± 0.9 versus 67% ± 0.5 in CABG, 88% ± 1.6 versus 67% ± 0.7 in THR). This difference was observed even in patients with preoperative Hct values over 44% in CABG (66% ± 1.9 versus 47% ± 1.5) or over 42% in THR (91% ± 3.3 versus 59% ± 1.8), and was also evident when blood loss was less than 500 mL in THR (81% ± 3.1 versus 42% ± 2.0).

In some hospitals, the results did not conform to this general pattern. For example, the probability of a patient being transfused in some hospitals was not significantly affected by the preoperative Hct value (see, for instance GBG and GRC in COLE), or by blood loss volume (see hospitals with high autotransfusion use, such as DB in THR).

After adjustment for age, gender and preoperative Hct, a patient's probability of being transfused still differed significantly among hospitals: the lowest and highest values ranged from 14% ± 4.4 to 72% ± 5.3 in COLE, from 24% ± 2.1 to 93% ± 1.4 in THR, from 62% ± 1.2 to 89% ± 1.3 in CABG and from 60% ± 1.6 to 88% ± 1.6 in AAA. After further adjustment for blood loss, the probability of a patient being transfused still differed significantly among hospitals, ranging from 27% ± 6.8 to 70% ± 10.7 in COLE and from 37% ± 5.7 to 87% ± 4.6 in THR (Figure 0.15). In the remaining interventions there were too few records of blood loss for this analysis to be performed.

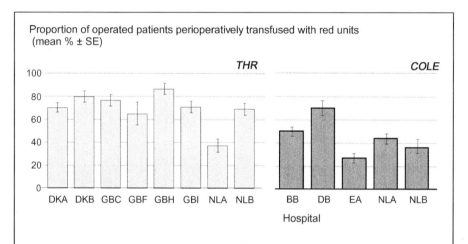

Fig 0.15. - Proportion of operated patients perioperatively transfused with red units in each hospital, after adjustment for age, gender, preoperative Hct, and blood loss in THR (total hip replacement) and COLE (right and left hemicolectomy). Each hospital is identified by a country code followed by a letter (e.g. NL (Netherlands), hospital A = NLA)

In-hospital outcomes of transfusion and surgery

Some outcomes of surgery and/or blood transfusion are reported in Table 0.5.

Table 0.5. Some in-hospital outcomes of blood transfusion and intervention

	Chole-cystectomy (CHOLE)	Right and left hemicolectomy (COLE)	Transurethral prostate resection (TURP)	Coronary artery bypass graft (CABG)	Abdominal aorta aneurysmectomy (AAA)	Total hip replacement (THR)
Median Hct value in patients transfused with red units, % last[1] available before discharge	34 (−)	35 (31-40)	34 (32-37)	34 (31-38)	34 (32-38)	33 (28-36)
Percentage of transfused patients showing a last[1] Hct value						
above 33%	51 (−)	64 (27-95)	51 (11-100)	51 (17-89)	58 (33-90)	43 (0-73)
under 24%		0.3 (0-10)	0.7 (0-7)	0.4 (0-2)	0.6 (0-11)	0.6 (0-8)
Reoperation for bleeding (% operated patients)	0.6 (0-7.7)	1.0 (0-6.5)	0.9 (0-5.7)	3.0 (0-9.7)	1.7 (0-12.5)	0.7 (0-7)
In-hospital crude mortality rate (% operated patients)	0.1 (0-1.2)	1.9 (0-16.7)	0.0 (0-1.8)	2.4 (0-16.7)	3.7 (0-25.0)	0.3 (0-3.4)
Postoperative length of hospital stay, median day number	7 (1-10)	12 (5-15)	5 (3-11)	10 (6-13)	11 (7-16)	14 (7-27)

Blank cells = 0.
In parentheses, the lowest-highest value observed among hospitals.
− = Value not calculated due to the small sample size.
[1] Recorded after all transfusions had been given, at a median of five to seven days after surgery, according to the procedure.

When the last available Hct before discharge is considered (i.e. the Hct recorded after all transfusions had been given, at a median of five to seven days after surgery depending on the procedure), it is seen that a substantial proportion of transfused patients showed a value falling outside the 24 to 33% interval, commonly considered appropriate for the postoperative period. [11, 12] In 16 hospitals, three quarters or more of transfused patients had a last Hct value higher than 33%, regardless of the surgical procedure. Of these, five were in Great Britain and seven in other central-northern European countries.

Complications of transfusion. Haemolytic transfusion reactions were reported by only three hospitals and concerned four patients.

Complications of surgery. These are described in the sections dealing with each procedure.

Documentation

Availability of data in the clinical record. The overall availability and the wide differences among hospitals in the recording of preoperative Hct value, perioperative blood loss and duration of surgery are illustrated in Figure 0.16.

A record of Hct was more often found for the day of surgery or one day before or after (Figures 0.17 and 0.18).

The mean number of Hct records per operated patient was 2.1 in TURP, 2.3 in CHOLE, 3.8 in THR, 4.1 in COLE, 5.2 in CABG and 5.6 in AAA.

Comparison between clinical record and files of the transfusion service (Figure 0.19).

Preoperative request. In 51% of hospitals an equal number of patients was found in both clinical and transfusion service records. In 28% of the hospitals a number of patients were recorded only in the files of the transfusion service, and in the remaining 21% only in the clinical records.

Allogeneic transfusion. The above values were 47, 9 and 44% respectively.

Adverse events of blood transfusion. A transfusion complication was documented in only 12 hospitals and, except for one of these, the information was more frequently found in the clinical records.

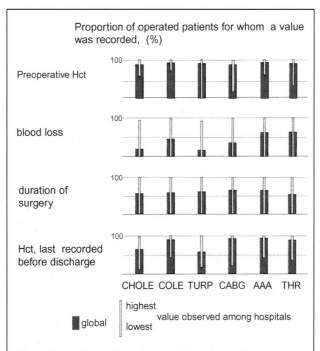

Fig 0.16. - Proportion of operated patients for whom at least one value of preoperative hematocrit (Hct), blood loss, duration of surgery and last Hct was found in the clinical record in CHOLE (laparotomic cholecystectomy), COLE (right and left hemicolectomy), TURP (transurethral prostatectomy), CABG (coronary artery bypass graft) and THR (total hip replacement)

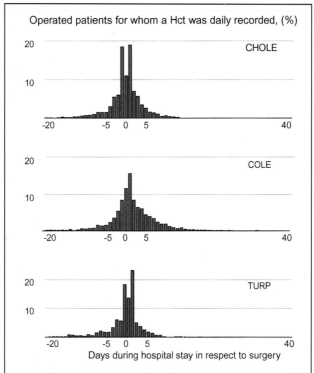

Operated patients for whom a Hct was daily recorded, (%)

Fig 0.17. - Proportion of operated patients for whom a Hct value was daily recorded during the hospital stay in CHOLE (cholecystectomy), COLE (right and left hemicolectomy) and transurethral prostatectomy (TURP)

Preoperative requests to the transfusion service

To evaluate the appropriateness of preoperative requests in relation to transfusion, CHOLE and TURP, procedures that seldom require red unit transfusion, were taken into consideration. Requests were aggregated into two groups according to whether the request was for the supply of red units or for Type and Screen (T&S). A request to supply blood requires the laboratory to determine ABO and Rh group, to perform a screening for red cell alloantibodies, to crossmatch the requested number of units and allocate them to a reserved inventory. A request for T&S does not require any crossmatch or unit allocation; a simplified version of donor-recipient compatibility is performed in case blood is needed. Figure 0.20 shows that the majority of the hospitals used T&S for both CHOLE and TURP, with the exception of hospitals from Belgium and Denmark, in which supply of red units was requested. Furthermore, the ratio between the proportion of operated patients with a request to that of operated patients ultimately transfused exceeded 10 in CHOLE, and four in TURP, with a large variability among hospitals (Figure 0.20).

Table 0.6 shows profiles of the patients for whom blood was and was not preoperatively ordered in both CHOLE and TURP. The two patient sub-sets show similarities for age, gender (CHOLE) and preoperative Hct.

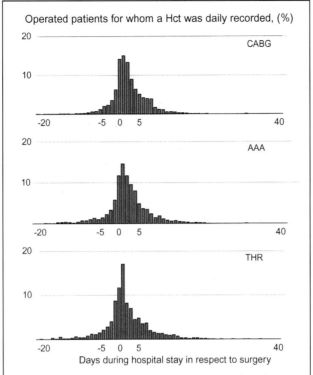

Fig 0.18. - Proportion of operated patients for whom a Hct value was daily recorded during the hospital stay in CABG (coronary artery bypass graft), AAA (abdominal aortic aneurysmectomy) and THR (total hip replacement)

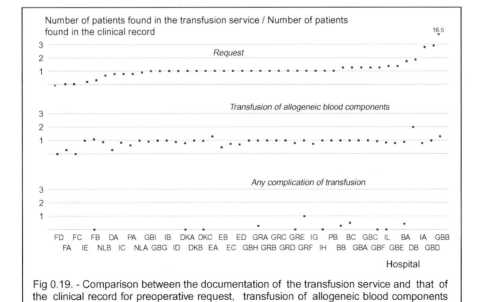

Fig 0.19. - Comparison between the documentation of the transfusion service and that of the clinical record for preoperative request, transfusion of allogeneic blood components and complications of transfusion

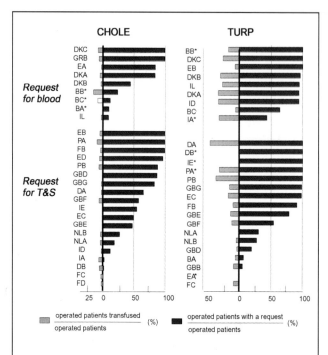

Fig 0.20. - Comparison between the proportion of operated patients for whom a request was made (right part of each figure) and that of patients ultimately transfused with blood (left part of each figure) in each hospital, for CHOLE (cholecystectomy) and TURP (transurethral prostatectomy.
* indicates hospitals enrolling less than 20 patients

Table 0.6. Some characteristics of patients for whom a preoperative request was and was not performed

	Patients		95% confidence interval of the difference
	with a preoperative request	without	
CHOLE			
Patient number	528	976	
Age, years[1]	58 ± 17	55 ± 16	− 1.30 to − 4.70
Percentage of males	33	32	− 5 to 3
Hct pretransfusion, %[1]	40 ± 4.7	40 ± 4.1	− 0.9 to 1.9
percentage of patients with	87	88	
TURP			
Patient number	677	513	
Age, years[1]	72 ± 9	71 ± 8	− 0.01 to − 1.90
Hct pretransfusion, %[1]	42 ± 5.1	42 ± 4.7	− 0.57 to − 0.57
percentage of patients with	88	92	

[1] Means ± SD

38

Preoperative requests ascertained from the files of the hospital transfusion services

For all the surgical procedures, a total of 19 371 red units were requested for 5 100 patients (71% of operated patients) and 2 081 units of plasma for 580 patients (8% of operated patients).

Allogeneic whole blood was requested for 25% of those patients for whom red units were ordered. This proportion ranged from 14 to 39% according to the surgical procedure, and from 0 to 100% according to the hospital (Figure 0.21).

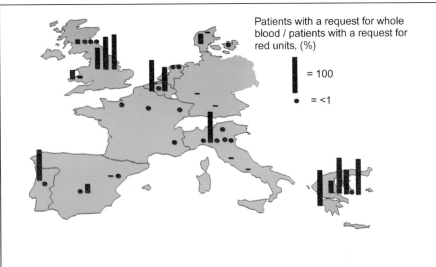

Patients with a request for whole blood / patients with a request for red units, (%)

| = 100

• = <1

Fig 0.21. - Request for whole blood in each hospital, regardless of the surgical procedure. *Source: files of the transfusion service*

Requests were submitted one (hinges: 1-2) day before surgery, irrespective of the surgical procedure; among different hospitals, orders were made from one day (hinges: 1-1) to four days before (hinges: 2-7), median values.

Figure 0.22 shows that in nearly one third of cases it was impossible to determine the status of the persons signing the blood request. Surgeons signed the majority (52%) of forms.

Requests of red units reported a preoperative Hct value in 22% of patients, this value ranging from 15 to 30% according to the surgical procedure, and from 0 to 100% according to the hospital.

The T&S procedure (Figure 0.23) was used in 28 of 43 hospitals (65%). The hospitals in Belgium and Denmark were among those not using it.

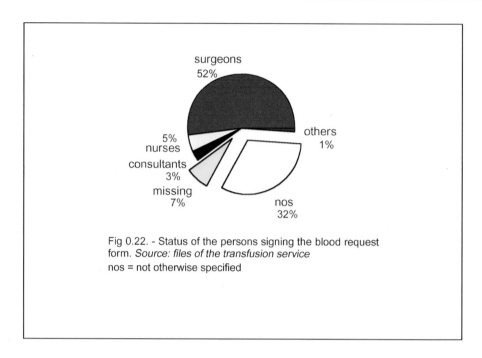

Fig 0.22. - Status of the persons signing the blood request form. *Source: files of the transfusion service*
nos = not otherwise specified

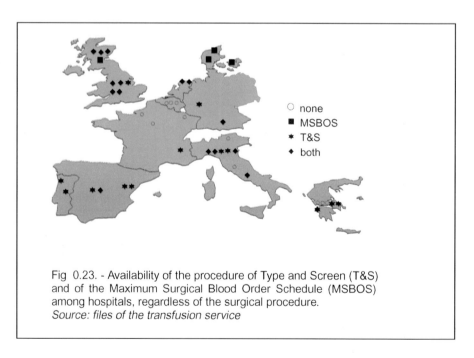

Fig 0.23. - Availability of the procedure of Type and Screen (T&S) and of the Maximum Surgical Blood Order Schedule (MSBOS) among hospitals, regardless of the surgical procedure. *Source: files of the transfusion service*

The preoperative request is usually defined by a locally developed maximum surgical blood order schedule, or MSBOS. This is a list of surgical procedures showing the number of units to be requested preoperatively. This rather standard procedure was found in only 19 of the 43 hospitals (44%). Hospitals from Belgium, France, Greece and Portugal did not use a MSBOS.

Part II
Individual surgical procedures

1.0. Laparotomic cholecystectomy (CHOLE) for cholelithiasis

Cholecystectomy is the definitive treatment for patients with symptomatic gallstones. Its frequency is second only to appendectomy. The male to female ratio is usually 1:3 at age 50, afterwards 1:1.5. The mortality rate is < 0.5%, and < 0.1% in individuals aged less than 50 years. Changes to laparoscopic procedures should decrease demands on blood transfusion.

Case report forms were available from 1 504 patients in 28 hospitals and 10 countries: 797 (53%) in 17 hospitals in six central-northern European countries and 707 (47%) in 11 hospitals in four Mediterranean countries (Figure 1.1).

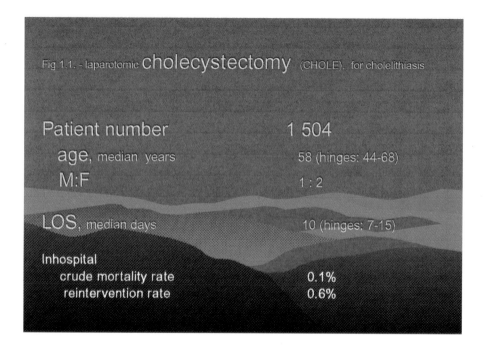

Fig 1.1. - laparotomic cholecystectomy (CHOLE), for cholelithiasis

Patient number	1 504
age, median years	58 (hinges: 44-68)
M:F	1 : 2
LOS, median days	10 (hinges: 7-15)
Inhospital	
crude mortality rate	0.1%
reintervention rate	0.6%

I. Patient data and some variables related to surgery

Table 1.1 reports, by hospital, the number, age and gender of patients along with the values of some variables related to surgery. Among hospitals, the M:F ranged from 1:1.4 to 1:3, and median age from 47 to 63 years.

A preoperative Hct value was available in 87% of patients. The median value was 40% (hinges: 38-43%).

Of operated patients, 57% received an anticoagulant drug (low-dose heparin in nearly all cases). In approximately half of the recipients low-dose heparin was given after surgery, in a quarter

Table 1.1. CHOLE: patient data and some variables related to surgery

	IE	EC	ID	FB	EB	ED	PB	PA	IL	DKA	GRB	GBD	GBE	FD	DA	GBG	EA	FC	NLB	GBF	BA*	BC*	IA	NLA	DKB	DB	DKC	BB*
Patient number	31	59	95	45	58	33	43	112	59	38	84	48	55	64	35	72	32	57	68	92	11	9	101	44	25	61	60	13
Age																												
median years	54	55	60	55	59	62	60	60	61	47	63	54	54	60	67	55	63	60	55	57	56	71	59	56	53	49	55	59
range	26-79	21-91	15-87	23-92	30-87	32-82	25-78	24-91	19-82	22-81	22-85	24-81	18-80	21-91	27-85	19-87	23-91	21-86	22-84	15-84	28-80	32-85	18-87	24-89	26-83	22-81	24-88	49-79
M:F ratio	0.3	0.6	0.4	0.3	0.7	0.4	0.6	0.4	0.4	0.5	0.5	0.4	0.3	0.5	0.7	0.5	0.4	0.5	0.5	0.5	0.8	0.1	0.4	0.7	0.3	0.6	0.3	0.8
Preoperative Hct																												
% Po with	100	57	74	100	89	79	95	92	75	87	95	71	87	86	100	92	78	96	98	94	91	100	91	98	84	79	85	100
%, median value	40	40	40	39	38	40	41	40	38	40	41	40	41	41	40	39	38	42	41	41	41	37	39	41	39	42	40	39
range	32-49	35-53	28-50	30-50	28-52	27-50	30-51	26-48	31-49	31-47	30-51	36-49	33-48	33-49	33-47	31-49	12-54	28-52	36-48	32-50	37-51	34-40	21-53	30-52	33-49	30-52	30-50	35-45
Drugs[1]																												
% Po	3.2	88	4	96	69		23	37	93	8	2	83	94	87	100	7	87	75	100	89	91	11	33	100	12	100	78	15
Anaesthesia																												
regional or combined % Po			8		3						11		2						1	4				23	8	2	5	
Duration of surgery																												
% Po with	100	100	15	80	100	100	100	63		97	46	73	62			67	100		75	62	82	89	27	86	80		100	61
median minutes	45	140	60	72	105	60	120	90		95	110	120	70			80	130		50	70			110	92	70		90	
range	30-60	60-190	45-120	30-150	55-210	60-135	60-360	45-160		50-190	60-215	40-250	30-150			40-200	70-140		20-110	30-170			45-205	30-200	45-145		45-270	
Blood loss																												
(i) perioperative																												
% Po with	42									58					43	10	44	60	46	5		44	7.0	27	76	44	95	61
median L	0.05									0.17					0.3	•	0.13	0.07	0.15	•		•	•	0.3	0.15	0.2	0.25	•
range	0.0-0.1									0.0-0.7					0.1-1.1		0.0-0.3	0.0-1.5	0.0-0.5					0.0-0.7	0.1-0.4	0.0-0.8	0.0-1.1	
(ii) postoperative																												
% Po with	61		8	100		2						2	27		1	1	22	65	13	50	91	89	1	29		23		69
median L	0.0		0.0	0.1		•						•	0.1		•	•	0.0	0.0	0.1	0.1	0.1	0.1	•	0.1		0.1		0.1
range	0.0-0.5		0.0-2.3	0.0-0.3		0.0-1.4						0.0-1.2	0.0-1.2		0.0-1.5		0.0-1.5	0.0-0.3	0.0-0.3	0.0-0.3	0.0-0.3		0.0-0.5	0.0-0.5		0.0-0.5		0.0-0.6

Po = operated patients.

• = not calculated due to the small sample size.

[1] Anticoagulants, except for two patients in two hospitals (BA, DB) who also received a haemostatic drug.

Hospital code and * = less than 20 patients.

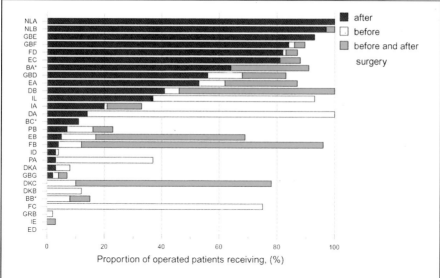

Fig 1.2. - CHOLE: anticoagulant administration by time in respect to surgery at each hospital

before surgery, and in the remaining quarter both before and after surgery. Figure 1.2 shows the great variability among hospitals both in the percentage of recipients and time of administration. In the hospitals of some countries (Great Britain, The Netherlands), low-dose heparin was given mainly after surgery.

General anaesthesia was used in the great majority of patients.

Information on duration of surgery was available in 56% of patients from 23 of 28 hospitals. The median duration was 90 (hinges: 60-130) minutes. Median values differed among hospitals by a factor of three, the minimum value being 45 minutes and the maximum 140 minutes. It is not known if differences in the duration of surgery reflected true differences in time or in the modalities of recording.

Perioperative blood loss was available in 20% of patients from 17 of 28 hospitals. The median volume was 0.2 L (hinges: 0.1-0.3). Of operated patients, 5% were reported to bleed 1 to 2.5 L (Figure 1.3). Information on postoperative blood loss was available in 18% of patients from 17 hospitals and the median volume was 0.08 L (hinges: 0.04-0.15).

II. Transfusion data

Table 1.2 shows, by hospital, the percentage of patients receiving each product and the amount of product per recipient. Less than 20% of patients were transfused with any product in any of the hospitals, with the exception of five (BA, BB, BC, NLA, DB), where albumin and/or artificial colloids were administered to up to two thirds of the patients. In hospitals of three countries (Great Britain, Belgium, Portugal) the same kind of products were used.

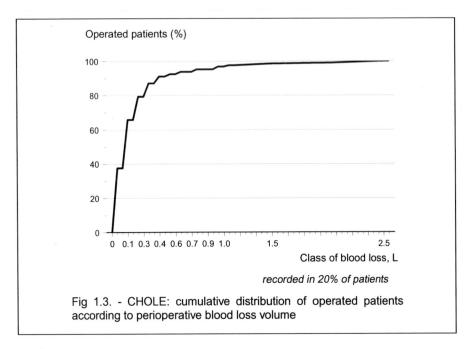

Fig 1.3. - CHOLE: cumulative distribution of operated patients according to perioperative blood loss volume

II.1.0. *Red units*

Of 1 504 patients (3.8%), 58 received 160 red units in 23 out of 28 hospitals. The percentage of patients transfused varied among hospitals from 0 to 8.3, without important differences between the two broad geographic areas.

In transfused patients, the median number of units was two (hinges: 2-3). Of operated patients, 0.3% received a number of red units greater than four (Figure 1.4).

II.1.1. *Autologous PABD units* were transfused to two patients in two hospitals (EA, DB).

II.1.2. *Whole blood*

Of allogeneic red units, 9% were used as whole blood in three hospitals (DKA, GBF, GRB), 6% being in one hospital (GBF).

II.2.0. *Plasma*

Twenty-two patients (1.5%) received 70 plasma units in 10 of 28 hospitals. Five patients (23% of those transfused) received one unit, nine (41%) two units, and the remaining eight patients (36%) 3 to 16 units.

In all 41% of plasma recipients were in one hospital (PA), whereas 63% of the units were used in two hospitals (GRB, PA). Fourteen patients were transfused with plasma only, while the remaining eight also received red units, seven of whom on the same day (hospitals IA, PA, PB).

Table 1.2. CHOLE: transfusion data

	IE	EC	ID	FB	EB	ED	PB	PA	IL	DKA	GRB	GBD	GBE	FD	DA	GBG	EA	FC	NLB	GBF	BA*	BC*	IA	NLA	DKB	DB	DKC	BB*
Red units																												
patients																												
transfused/operated (%)		1.7	3.1		5.2	6.1	7.0	4.5	3.4	5.3	4.8				2.9	2.8	3.1	3.5	4.4	6.5			6.9	2.3	4	4.9	8.3	7.7
Plasma																												
patients																												
transfused/operated (%)				4.4			4.6	8.0			2.4			1.6			3.1						2.0	2.3		1.6		7.7
Platelets																												
patients																												
transfused/operated (%)								0.9															1.0					
Albumin																												
patients																												
administered/operated (%)									1.7	5.3	1.2										36.4	66.7	15.8	9.1	12	3.3	3.3	38.5
grams per patient administered																												
median									•	•	•										•		16		21	•	•	•
hinges																							11-39		13-21			
Lyophilized plasma																												
patients																												
transfused/operated (%)											1.2																	
Colloids																												
patients																												
administered/operated (%)												6.2	9.1	12.5	20.0	8.3	3.1	5.2	19.1	5.4	36.4	11.1	1.0	31.8	8.0	59.0	16.7	15.4
L per patient administered																												
median													•	0.5	0.5	•	•	•	0.5	•	•	•	•	0.5	•	0.5	0.5	•
hinges														0.5-0.5	0.5-0.5				0.5-0.5					0.5-0.5		0.5-0.5	0.5-0.5	

Hospitals are aggregated according to products used.
• = not calculated due to the small sample size.
Hospital code and * = less than 20 patients.
' Use of autotransfusion.

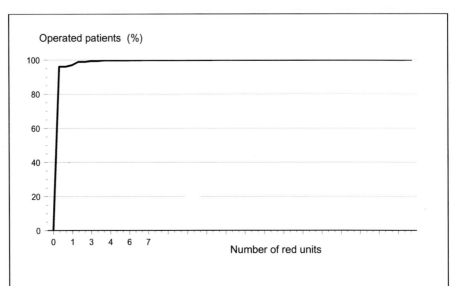

Fig 1.4. - CHOLE: cumulative distribution of operated patients according to the number of red units transfused

Of 70 plasma units, 69 were allogeneic; of them, eight were apheresis units (hospital IA), four were liquid (hospitals NLA, PB) and the remaining 57 were fresh frozen units.

II.3.0. *Albumin*

Forty-five patients (3%) received 1 430 g of albumin in 11 of the 28 hospitals, eight of them being of central-northern European countries.

33% of all albumin recipients and 53% of all the total quantity used were observed in Belgian hospitals although they provided only 2% of CHOLE patients. The percentage of patients receiving albumin was similar between the two broad geographic areas, after exclusion of patients from Belgian hospitals due to the small size of the patient sample.

II.4.0. *Artificial colloids*

In all 122 patients (8%) were transfused with 70.9 L of artificial colloids in 17 hospitals; of them, nine used gelatin, three dextran, and the remaining five a mixture of various colloids (Figure 1.5). The great majority of hospitals using artificial colloids were in the central-northern European area. Here, in fact, the percentage of artificial colloid recipients was higher than that of the Mediterranean area (RR = 101 (43 to 239)). Such RR values were due to the occurrence of only two patients receiving colloids in hospitals of the Mediterranean area. The median administered volume was 0.5 L (hinges: 0.5-0.5).

35% of artificial colloids recipients and one third of the total volume administered were used in the two German hospitals.

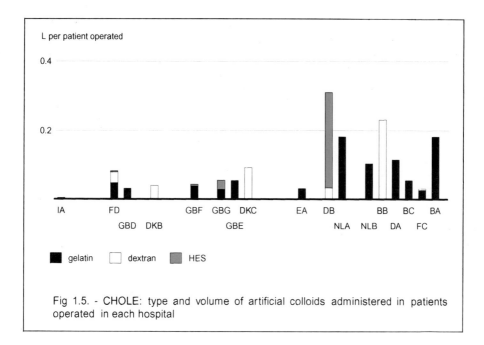

Fig 1.5. - CHOLE: type and volume of artificial colloids administered in patients operated in each hospital

The great variability among hospitals in the use of the studied products and their combinations are shown in Figure 1.6 and that among hospitals aggregated by country in Figure 1.7.

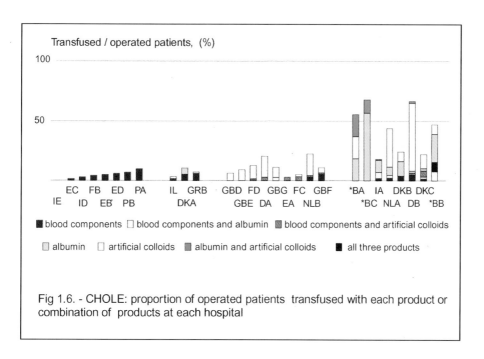

Fig 1.6. - CHOLE: proportion of operated patients transfused with each product or combination of products at each hospital

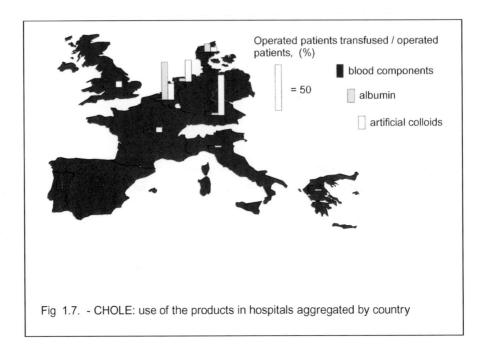

Fig 1.7. - CHOLE: use of the products in hospitals aggregated by country

III. Reasons for perioperative transfusion documented in the medical record

III.1. *Red units*

Of the recipients, 30% had a documented reason; this proportion ranged from 0 to 100% according to the hospital (Figure 1.8).

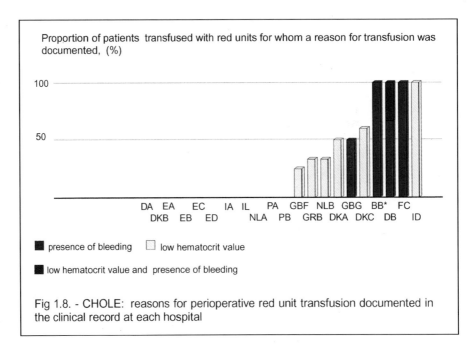

Fig 1.8. - CHOLE: reasons for perioperative red unit transfusion documented in the clinical record at each hospital

III.2. *Plasma*

Reasons were found in four patients (25%) from three hospitals (BB, FD, GRB).

III.3. *Albumin*

Reasons were found in two patients (4%) from two hospitals (BB, DB).

III.4. *Artificial colloids*

Reasons were found in 33 recipients (28%), 23 of them in one hospital (DB).

IV. Variables associated with red unit transfusion

IV.1. *Transfused versus untransfused patients*

A high age, a low preoperative Hct value and a high blood loss volume (Table 1.3) characterized transfused patients, even after exclusion of deaths and reinterventions. Transfused patients also showed a longer post-surgical LOS. It is of note that half of the transfused patients had a last Hct value over 33%.

Table 1.3. CHOLE: comparison between patients transfused and not transfused with allogeneic red units during the hospital stay

| | Patients | | 95% confidence interval of |
	transfused	not transfused	the difference[2]
Number of patients	56	1 446	
age,[1] years	*67 (58-79)*	*57 (44-68)*	*− 14.2 to − 5.8*
M:F	0.60	0.47	− 7 to 18
Preoperative Hct value,[1] %	*36 (31-41)*	*40 (38-43)*	*2.8 to 5.2*
% patients with	84	88	
Anaesthesia, regional and/or combined, % Po	7.1	2.6	
Anticoagulants, % Po	55	57	
Duration of surgery, minutes[1]	90 (60-122)	90 (60-130)	
% patients with	57	56	
Blood loss, mL[1]			
perioperative	*0.47 (0.2-1.0)*	*0.17 (0.1-0.3)*	*0.30 to 0.82*[3]
% patients with	32	19	
Red units per patient transfused[1]	2 (2-3)		
Percentage of patients transfused with			
plasma	14.3		
albumin	14.3	2.6	
artificial colloids	17.9	7.6	
Reintervention for bleeding, % Po	10.7	0.14	
In-hospital crude mortality rate, % Po	1.79	0.07	
Hct value, %,[1]			
last available before discharge	33 (30-37)	37 (34-40)	
% patients with	89	64	
Hospital stay, days[1]	18 (10-25)	9 (7-14)	
before surgery	2 (1-12)	2 (1-5)	
after surgery	10 (7-13)	7 (5-9)	

Po = patients operated.

[1] Median (hinges).

[2] Between patients not transfused and transfused with allogeneic units, after exclusion of deaths and reinterventions.

[3] Performed on ln values.

Note: **significant differences are shown in bold italics.**

IV.2. *Preoperative transfusion*

Seven patients (0.5%) were transfused preoperatively; five were females and two males. They were aged 67 to 89 years (median 79), values falling above the upper quartile of patient distribution by age. Their Hct value before transfusion (available in five patients) ranged from 21 to 32% (median 23%) and after transfusion of two units (mean, median) from 26 to 38% (median 29%). One of these patients was subsequently reoperated for bleeding and one died.

IV.3. *Postoperative transfusion*

Twelve patients (0.8%) were postoperatively transfused. Their median age was 75 years (range: 33 to 83) and the M:F ratio was 5:7. Of them, three were reoperated for bleeding and one died. Pretransfusion Hct values (recorded in five patients) ranged from 21 to 32% and post-transfusion Hct values (recorded in two patients) were 29 and 38%.

V. In-hospital outcomes of transfusion and surgery

Table 1.4 shows some outcome variables. The last Hct value was recorded in 65% of operated patients at a median number of two days (hinges: 1-4) after surgery. The median value was 37% (hinges: 34-40%). In all hospitals except one (EA), the median Hct value was higher than 33%.

In patients transfused with red units, the last Hct was recorded (after all transfusions were given) in half, at a median number of five days (hinges: 3-8) after surgery. The median value was 34% (hinges: 30-38%). No patient had a Hct value lower than 24% (Part I, Table 0.5).

In operated patients the decrease from preoperative to last available Hct value was $-3.1\% \pm 3.8$ after transfusion of 0.1 ± 0.8 red units per patient (means ± SD). The lowest and highest Hct fall observed among hospitals was $-1.3\% \pm 3.5$ (Figure 1.9) and $-5.5\% \pm 4.8$ (means ± SD), respectively, with no units transfused.

Complications of surgery

Reoperation for bleeding (Table 1.5) was four times more frequent in females than in males. In reoperated patients, preoperative and last Hct values fell both below the lower quartile of the relative distribution, while perioperative and postoperative blood loss, and postoperative LOS fell above the upper quartile of their distributions.

Complications of blood transfusion

No complications were reported.

Median LOS before surgery was two days (hinges: 1-6) and after surgery seven days (hinges: 5-9). Preoperative LOS (Figure 1.10) was shorter in hospitals of central-northern Europe than in hospitals of the Mediterranean area, namely one (hinges: 1-2) versus four days (hinges: 2-10), median values.

Table 1.4. CHOLE: some outcome variables

	IE	EC	ID	FB	EB	ED	PB	PA	IL	DKA	GRB	GBD	GBE	FD	DA	GBG	EA	FC	NLB	GBF	BA*	BC*	IA	NLA	DKB	DB	DKC	BB*
Last Hct																												
% Po with	81	36	88	71	65	97	49	61	93	68	61	12	53	23	66	42	22	65	90	66	91	89	83	66	84	95	65	92
%, median value	38	38	37	36	37	40	37	36	35	37	39	37	36	36	37	36	31	38	38	37	39	35	37	37	33	39	35	35
range	31-45	33-49	27-49	29-44	25-44	28-50	25-45	24-45	28-45	29-48	30-47	33-38	31-46	25-45	25-44	27-44	23-49	28-50	30-46	19-50	31-43	30-41	24-48	25-49	28-43	28-49	25-46	26-42
Reoperation																												
% Po			1.0			3.0					1.2	2.1					3.1			1.1					4.0	1.6		7.7
Mortality																												
% Po											1.2												1.0					
LOS																												
median day number	10	9	12	12	16	11	21	13	12	5	10	2	6	7	13	7	11	9	9	6	12	16	15	10	9	6	9	9
range	6-25	5-25	4-57	6-27	5-48	4-41	6-49	3-68	7-22	2-29	4-50	0-11	3-14	4-37	6-34	3-35	4-36	3-33	5-29	3-28	8-19	9-25	4-63	6-29	5-22	2-19	4-30	1-11

No complications of allogeneic or autologous blood transfusion were reported.
Po = patients operated.
Hospital code and * = less than 20 patients.

Table 1.5. CHOLE: complications of surgery

	Hospital number	Patient number	Age, years [1]	Gender M:F [1]	Hct, % preoperative [1]	Perioperative blood loss, L [1]	Postoperative blood loss, L [1]	Red units per patient [1]	Last Hct, % [1]	Postoperative LOS days [1]	Death: days after surgery [1]
Reoperation for bleeding:	9	9	48 (27-80)	1:8	36 (30-43)	0.3 (0.1-0.5)	. (0.8-1.5)	2 (1-7)	. (30-38)	16 (7-27)	
recorded in	9/28	9/1 504			6/9	5/9	3/9	7/9	4/9		
deaths	2	2	74-80	1:1	32-32			0-27			4-10
recorded in	2/28	2/1 504			2/2	0/2	0/2	1/2	0/2		

. = not calculated due to the small sample size.
[1] Median (range).

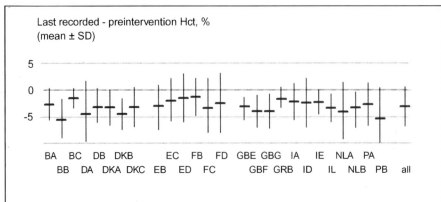

Fig 1.9. - CHOLE: fall of hematocrit value in operated patients. Only hospitals are reported where Hct values were recorded in at least eight patients

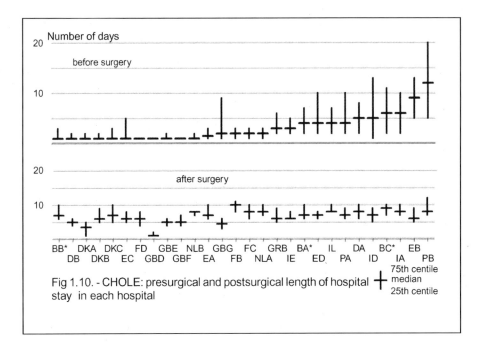

Fig 1.10. - CHOLE: presurgical and postsurgical length of hospital stay in each hospital

VI. Costs

Overall estimated cost due to the product use per operated patient accounted for ECU 11 and that due to preoperative request for ECU 5. Costs for product use ranged from ECU 0 to 90 according to the hospital (Figure 1.11) and those for preoperative request from ECU 0 to 10.

The impact of albumin use on the overall costs, although moderated, in the three Belgian hospitals is evident.

A summary of the findings is reported in Table 1.6.

Table 1.6. CHOLE: summary of main findings

			in hospitals (of 28)
Preoperative request			
percentage of operated patients with		50.6 (0-100)	26
MSBOS			9
T&S			19
Red units			
percentage of patients transfused			
	total	3.8 (0-8)	21
	allogeneic	3.7 (0-8)	
	autologous	0.1 (0-3)	2
factors implied:	transfused vs. untransfused patients		
age, years (median)		67 vs. 57	
preoperative Hct, % (median)		36 vs. 40	
perioperative blood loss, mL (median)		475 vs. 175	
reinterventions (% patients)		10.7 vs. 0.14	
deaths (% patients)		1.79 vs. 0.07	
last Hct, % (median)		33 vs. 37	
fall in Hct value, mean ± SD (last - preoperative Hct), %		-3.1 ± 3.8	
whole blood use (percentage of red units used as whole blood)		9 (0-67)	3
Plasma			
percentage of patients transfused		1 (0-8)	10
Albumin			
percentage of patients receiving		3 (0-67)	11
Artificial colloids			
percentage of patients receiving		8 (0-59)	17
percentage of colloids used as			
gelatin		53 (0-100)	13
dextran		19 (0-100)	6
HES		28 (0-89)	4
Other variables			
administration of low-dose heparin (% patients)			
before		11 (0-100)	20
after		32 (0-100)	21
before and after surgery		14 (0-82)	14
LOS, median day number			
before surgery		2 (1-12)	
after surgery		7 (1-10)	

In parentheses the lowest-highest value observed among hospitals.

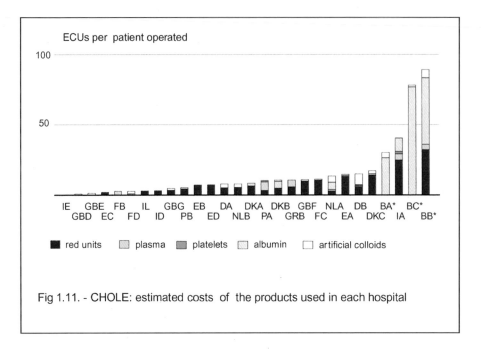

Fig 1.11. - CHOLE: estimated costs of the products used in each hospital

VII. Comments on CHOLE

The most frequent aspect of transfusion practice in CHOLE was represented by the preoperative request. It in fact involved 51% operated patients, a proportion much higher than that of any product recipient: 8% received artificial colloids, 4% red units, 3% albumin. Preoperative request creates laboratory work and costs and in many cases also requires the removal of red units from the free inventory available for other patients. In surgical procedures such as cholecystectomy, that are frequently performed and have a very low probability of transfusion, the costs and benefits of the preoperative request should be re-evaluated. If we estimate that 312 000 laparotomic CHOLE interventions are performed each year in the 12 countries of the European Union, and consider only the costs of conventional pre-transfusion tests (about ECU 10/patient), ECU 1.57 million are spent yearly in the 12 EU countries for a procedure which provides no benefits for about 95% of the operated patients.

In the Sanguis hospitals, the preoperative assessment overestimated the probability of patients needing red unit transfusion since blood or T&S requested were made for 10 times more patients than were eventually transfused. There was no evidence that patients were selected by risk factor for preoperative request, since age and preoperative Hct were similar for patients for whom a preoperative request was or was not made. Practical factors such as the distance between the surgical unit and the transfusion service may in some cases require special steps to ensure the availability of blood in an emergency. However, the finding that standard measures, such as MSBOS and T&S, were only adopted by some hospitals, suggests that rational cost reduction has received little attention. Closer attention to identifying those patients more likely to require transfusion and the proximity of an active transfusion service should make it possible to safely minimize preoperative requests. This could provide significant financial savings without jeopardizing patients.

Sanguis confirmed, from a large patient sample of broad origin and from many hospitals, the low probability of transfusion (3.8%). The patients who did receive transfusion were older, had lower preoperative Hct values and higher blood loss than untransfused patients. These factors were also documented in the medical record, although in only a minority of patients. Transfusion in many cases resulted in a final post-transfusion Hct higher than generally considered necessary, [11, 12] indicating that clinicians may believe that higher Hct values are desirable, at least in elderly patients.

Autotransfusion in CHOLE was almost never used, in accordance with the views of most authors. [13-15]

The high use of whole blood in one hospital in Great Britain may be assumed to be a local factor in the organization of blood supplies, as suggested by similar findings for other surgical procedures in that location.

A limited use of plasma, usually in doses too small to have a haemostatic effect, was observed, principally in one hospital.

There were great differences in the use of albumin and artificial colloids among hospitals, even within a country, ranging from 0 to 67% and from 0 to 59%, respectively, of patients operated. The highest proportion of albumin and artificial colloid recipients was observed in the Belgian and German hospitals, respectively. Such variability may in part reflect differences in the availability of the individual products, as suggested by regional or national trends in use, or clinical preference, as suggested by use within the same country where it would be expected that health-care organization and access to the products could be fairly uniform.

The data suggest that there are differences among hospitals in other aspects of practice, such as anticoagulant administration, and preoperative LOS, a variable that is often affected by hospital organization. The long preoperative LOS for all procedures in hospitals of the Mediterranean area (especially certain hospitals, such as PB and ID, where preoperative LOS was among the longest observed) also suggested that there are important organizational differences.

2.0. Transurethral resection of the prostate (TURP) for benign prostatic hyperplasia

Benign prostatic hyperplasia (BPH) usually presents clinically after age 50, the incidence increasing with age but as many as two thirds of men aged 40 to 49 years demonstrate evidence of the disease. It is estimated that one in 10 men living until age 80 will require prostatectomy for relief of urinary obstruction. TURP is generally regarded as a safe and effective procedure in overcoming urinary obstruction when the prostate weight is less than 50 g. Mortality rate is usually in the range of 0.1 to 0.5%. The relative benefit of TURP versus open prostatectomy has recently been reassessed.

Case report forms were available from 1 190 patients in 26 hospitals and nine countries: 861 (72%) in 17 hospitals in six central-northern European countries and 329 (28%) in nine hospitals in three Mediterranean countries (Figure 2.1).

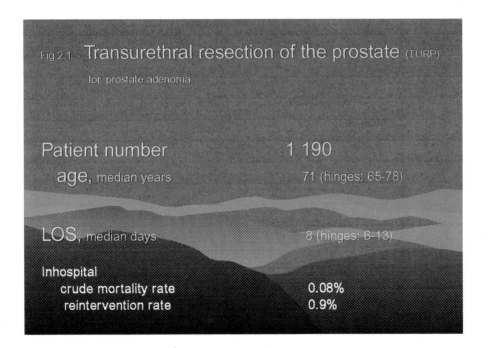

Fig 2.1 Transurethral resection of the prostate (TURP)
for prostate adenoma

Patient number	1 190
age, median years	71 (hinges: 65-78)
LOS, median days	8 (hinges: 6-13)
Inhospital	
crude mortality rate	0.08%
reintervention rate	0.9%

I. Patient data and some variables related to surgery

Table 2.1 shows, by hospital, the number and age of patients along with the values of some variables related to surgery. In nearly two thirds of the hospitals, patients were aged 71 to 75 years, and in the remaining third, 65 to 70 years (median values).

Preoperative Hct value was available in 90% of patients, the median value being 43% (hinges: 39 to 45%). In all hospitals the median value was 40% or higher.

Of operated patients, 34% received a drug acting on the coagulation system which in nearly all patients was an anticoagulant. Of the recipients, 15% were given an anticoagulant only before

Table 2.1. TURP: patient data and some variables related to surgery

	EA*	DB*	IE*	EB	EC	IL	PA*	ID	PB	DKA	GBD	BA	NLB	FC	GBF	GBE	GBG	NLA	BC	GBB	FB	BB*	DKC	DKB	IA*	DA
Patient number	1	7	11	60	59	62	13	74	33	59	30	54	50	55	53	66	73	39	67	35	104	12	60	62	16	35
Age, median years	•	65	65	71	70	75	70	68	66	73	69	69	71	65	71	69	73	72	70	71	71	73	73	72	59	74
Age, range		52-72	59-84	57-89	55-92	54-91	58-85	44-84	52-81	53-92	60-86	49-84	45-90	52-91	63-91	49-86	59-90	51-90	49-90	52-87	47-91	47-84	50-91	47-85	52-76	59-91
Preoperative Hct, % Po with	•	100	100	87	41	81	54	97	100	86	93	93	98	96	98	92	92	100	100	94	81	100	100	92	100	91
%, median value		43	46	43	43	43	45	44	44	41	43	43	43	43	44	42	42	43	44	45	41	40	41	42	42	41
range		39-49	39-49	28-56	28-54	29-56	23-45	31-52	28-57	30-50	31-49	30-53	35-51	18-51	28-54	32-51	27-52	33-51	33-52	35-55	20-55	30-47	32-53	29-50	34-47	28-51
Drugs[1], % Po	•	86		18	85	100	15	19	6	22	17	13	100	11	11	8	16	100	15	20	28	33	8	31	69	100
Anaesthesia, regional or combined, % Po	•	100	100	97	90	13	15	84	85	88	90	91	98	38	25	50	38	95	98	91	87	25	63	24		57
Duration of surgery, % Po with	•	100	100	95	98		38		100	71	100	67	74		51	65	66	64	81	60	85	58	98	74		
median minutes		40	75	75	190		150		60	55	60	62	45		45	60	40	65	50	45	45	80	50	70		
range		35-65	60-180	60-180	40-250		150-160		45-180	15-165	25-110	25-120	15-99		20-80	20-110	20-90	25-120	15-120	30-140	15-165	25-150	20-190	15-135		
Blood loss[2], perioperative, % Po with		14						3		81			92	9	2	4	5	3	1			8	38	74	19	46
median L		•						•		0.50			0.50	•	•	•	•	•	•			•	0.50	0.42	•	0.30
range										0.1-4.6			0.2-1.0										0.0-2.3	0.1-1.3		0.1-1.0

Po = patients operated.

[1] Only anticoagulants were administered.

[2] For 35 out of 1 190 patients (3%) — half of them in hospital ID — postoperative blood loss volumes were recorded, median volume 0.1 L, range 0.0-1.5.

• = not calculated due to the small sample size.

Hospital code and * = less than 20 patients.

surgery, 14% only after surgery, and 5% both before and after surgery. Before surgery the drug was aspirin/NSAID (9%) or low-dose heparin (6%); after surgery it was low-dose heparin (10%), coumarin (2%), or not specified (2%); and for those treated both before and after surgery the anticoagulant was low-dose heparin in nearly all cases. Figure 2.2 shows how hospitals differed in the percentage of drug recipients as well as in time of administration. Hospitals from Great Britain and Denmark tended to use anticoagulants mainly before surgery, those from the Netherlands after surgery, and those from Germany both before and after surgery.

Anaesthesia was regional in 66% of the cases, general in 32% and combined in 2%. Among hospitals, extremes were observed, with some hospitals using only general (IA) or regional anaesthesia (DB).

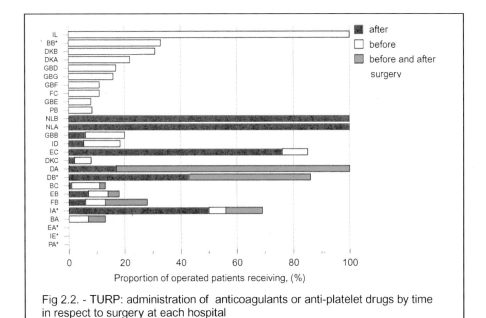

Fig 2.2. - TURP: administration of anticoagulants or anti-platelet drugs by time in respect to surgery at each hospital

Information on the duration of surgery was available in 61% of patients and about three quarters of the hospitals. The median value was 60 minutes (hinges: 40-90). The minimum and maximum of the median values observed between hospitals were 40 and 190 minutes, respectively. It is not known if interhospital diversities reflected true differences in time or different ways of recording the operation time.

In none of the surgical procedures was the information related to blood loss as poor as in TURP. Only three hospitals reported blood loss for more than half of the patients (DKA, DKB, NLB). The median value of perioperative blood loss (Figure 2.3) was 0.5 L (hinges: 0.3-0.6).

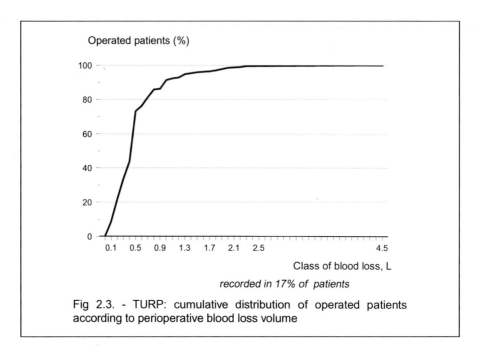

Fig 2.3. - TURP: cumulative distribution of operated patients according to perioperative blood loss volume

II. Transfusion data

Table 2.2 shows, by hospital, the percentage of patients receiving each product and the amount of product per recipient. The majority of the hospitals (with 20 or more operated patients) used blood components together with albumin and/or artificial colloids. Hospitals of nearly all countries differed in the type of products used.

II.1.0. *Red units*

Of 1 190 operated patients, 197 (16.5%) received 555 red units in 22 of 26 hospitals. The percentage of transfused patients varied greatly among hospitals: from 0 to 45%. In the hospitals of central-northern European countries the proportion of patients transfused was about one third less than in hospitals of the Mediterranean area (RR = 0.6 (0.5 to 0.8)).

In transfused patients, the median number of units was two (hinges: 2-3). Of operated patients, 2.2% (Figure 2.4) received more than four red units.

II.1.1. *Autologous transfusion*

Fourteen patients (1%) received 23 autologous red units in four (BB, DA, IA, PB) hospitals: eight patients 13 PABD units (DA, PB), four patients five PIH units (BB, IA) and two patients five IBS units (DA).

Table 2.2. TURP: transfusion data

	EA*	DB*	IE*	EB	EC	IL	PA*	ID	PB	DKA	GBD	BA	NLB	FC	GBF	GBE	GBG	NLA	BC	GBB	FB	BB*	DKC	DKB	IA*	DA
Red units																										
patients	[1]	–	–						[1]													[1]			[1]	[1]
transfused/operated (%)	6.7				16.9	25.8	30.8	32.4	33.3	32.2	3.3	3.7	4.0	9.1	11.3	13.6	15.1		6.0	8.6	9.6	16.7	25.0	29.0	31.2	45.7
units																										
per transfused patient																										
median				•	2	3.5	•	2	1	2	•	•	•	•	2.5	2	2		•	•	•	•	2	2	•	2
hinges					2-2	2-7.5		2-2	1-2	1-4					2-3	2-2	2-4						1-2	2-4		2-4
Plasma																										
patients																										
transfused/operated (%)							7.7	1.3	15.1	1.7		1.8	2.0				1.4				1.0		1.7		6.2	8.6
units																										
per transfused patient																										
median							•	•	1	•	•	•	•	•	•	•	•		•		•		•		•	•
hinges									1-1																	
Platelets																										
patients																										
transfused/operated (%)													2.0													
Albumin																										
patients																										
recipients/operated (%)										8.5								10.2	10.4	2.8	1.9	16.7	8.3	9.7	18.7	5.7
grams per administered patient																										
median										•								21	21	•	•	•	•	•	•	•
hinges																		21-21	21-21							
Colloids																										
patients																										
recipients/operated (%)											16.7	11.1	62.0	7.3	17.0	21.2	13.7	17.9	11.9	8.6	89.4	8.3	23.3	19.3	6.2	57.1
L per administered patient																										
median											0.5	0.5	0.5	•	0.5	0.5	0.5	0.5	0.5	•	0.5	•	0.5	0.5	•	0.5
hinges											0.5-0.5	0.5-0.5	0.5-0.5		0.5-0.5	0.5-0.5	0.5-1	0.5-0.5	0.5-0.5		0.5-0.5		0.5-0.5	0.5-0.5		0.5-0.5

Hospitals are aggregated according to products used.
• = not calculated due to the small sample size.
Hospital code and * = less than 20 patients.
[1] = use of autotransfusion.

63

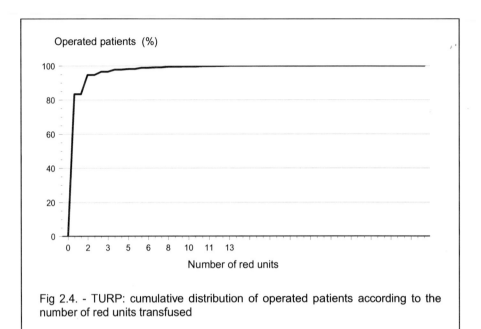

Fig 2.4. - TURP: cumulative distribution of operated patients according to the number of red units transfused

II.1.2. *Whole blood*

3% of allogeneic red units were used as whole blood, two hospitals (GBE, GBF) accounting for two thirds of all the whole blood used for TURP. In these hospitals whole blood represented 25 to 37% of all the red units transfused.

II.2.0. *Plasma*

In all 43 units of plasma were transfused to 17 patients (1%) in 11 hospitals, the median number of plasma units being two (hinges: 1-3). Nearly one third of plasma recipients were in PB. One third of all plasma units were transfused in DA.

Of 17 plasma recipients, 15 were also transfused with red units, 13 of them within the same 24-hour period.

Of 43 plasma units transfused, 31 were fresh frozen, eight liquid (DKA, PB), and four from apheresis (BB, IA).

II.3.0. *Albumin*

In 10 of 26 hospitals, 1 115 g of albumin were administered to 37 patients (3%). All recipients were from hospitals of central-northern Europe. Albumin was used to a maximum of 10% in any hospital. In recipients, the amount of albumin was 21 g (hinges: 21-38), median value. Half of all the administered albumin was given in the three Danish hospitals, DKA accounting for one fourth.

II.4.0. *Artificial colloids*

In all 145 L of artificial colloids were administered to 20% of operated patients from two thirds of the hospitals, all in central-northern Europe. While the percentage of colloid recipients varied greatly among hospitals, no variation was observed in the volume administered: in recipients, the median volume was in fact 0.5 L (hinges: 0.5-0.5).

60% of recipients were in three hospitals (FB, NLB, DA), FB accounting for 38% of the total quantity used.

Of 16 hospitals where colloids were used, eight used gelatin, three dextran, four both gelatin and HES, and one gelatin with dextran (Figure 2.5). In recipients, a median volume of 0.5 L was given, independent of the type of colloid.

The variety of products used in the various hospitals is shown in Figure 2.6 and in hospitals aggregated according to the country in Figure 2.7.

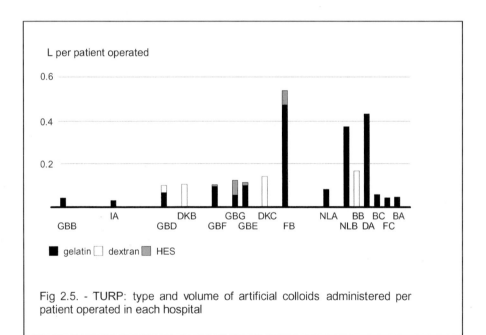

Fig 2.5. - TURP: type and volume of artificial colloids administered per patient operated in each hospital

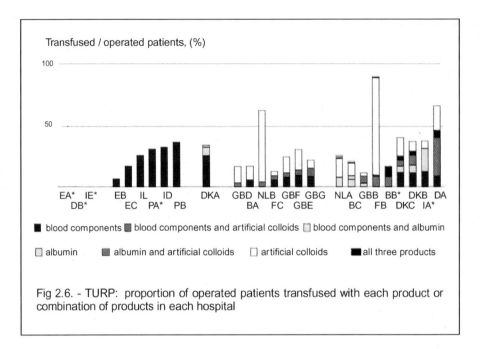

Fig 2.6. - TURP: proportion of operated patients transfused with each product or combination of products in each hospital

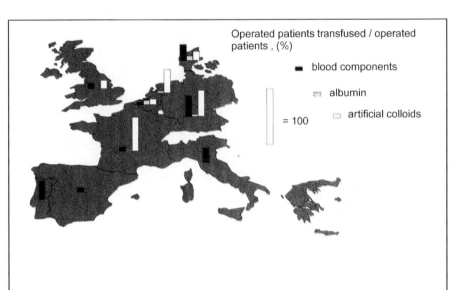

Fig 2.7. - TURP: use of the products in hospitals aggregated by country

III. Reasons for perioperative transfusion documented in the medical record

III.1. *Red units*

A reason was documented in 27% of transfused patients (Figure 2.8). Hospitals documenting were mainly those in the central-northern European area.

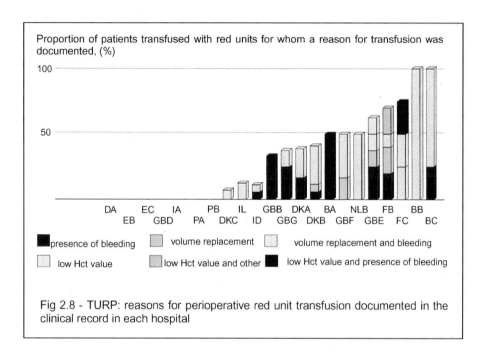

Fig 2.8 - TURP: reasons for perioperative red unit transfusion documented in the clinical record in each hospital

III.2. *Plasma*

Reasons were found in two patients (13%) from two hospitals (BA, DA).

III.3. *Albumin*

Reasons were found in two patients (5%) from two hospitals (BC, DKC).

III.4. *Artificial colloids*

Reasons were found in five patients (2%) from three hospitals (FB, FC, GBE).

IV. Variables associated with red unit transfusion

IV.1. *Transfused versus untransfused patients*

The profiles of patients transfused and not transfused with red units during the hospital stay are reported in Table 2.3. Patients transfused with allogeneic red units were slightly older than untransfused patients, had a lower preoperative Hct value, and a higher perioperative blood loss, even after exclusion of deaths and of reoperations. It is notable that in half of the transfused patients the last Hct value was higher than 33%.

The few patients transfused only with autologous blood were the youngest among the three patient groups. It may be that the absence of comorbid conditions made them appropriate candidates for PABD and PIH in given hospitals.

Table 2.3. TURP: profiles of patients transfused and not transfused with red units during the hospital stay

	Patients transfused			Patients not transfused	95% confidence interval of the difference[2]
	allogeneic	allogeneic and autologous	autologous		
Patient number	183	4	10	993	
Age, years[1]	*75 (69-80)*	. (56-75)	65 (64-78)	*70 (65-77)*	*−4 to −6*
Hct[1] preoperative, %	*40 (36-44)*	. (39-45)	41 (37-45)	*43 (40-46)*	*2.2 to 3.8*
Percentage of patients with	90	100	100	90	
Anaesthesia, regional and/or combined, % Po	60	25	80	69	
Anticoagulants, % Po	35	75	50	34	
Duration of surgery,[1] minutes	80 (60-120)	. (120-150)	70 (60-120)	60 (40-80)	
Percentage of patients with	54	50	60	63	
Blood loss,[1] L					
perioperative	*0.8 (0.5-1.1)*	.	.	*0.4 (0.2-0.5)*	*0.33 to 0.61*[3]
Percentage of patients with	32			14	
Red units per patient transfused[1]	3 (2-4)	. (4-5)	2 (2-2)		
Percentage of patients transfused with					
plasma	7.1	50.0			
albumin	13.1	75.0	10	0.9	
artificial colloids	26.2	50.0	30	18.6	
PABD, % patients		100	100		
Stated reason for transfusion, Percentage of patients transfused	30	25			
Reintervention for bleeding, % Po	4.37			0.3	
In-hospital crude mortality rate, % Po				0.1	
Last Hct,[1] %	33 (30-36)	. (28-33)	33 (28-36)	38 (34-41)	
Percentage of patients with	85	100	70	53	
Hospital stay,[1] day number	12 (8-19)	. (12-18)	18 (11-20)	7 (5-11)	
before surgery	4 (1-9)	. (1-8)	5 (4-11)	2 (1-5)	
after surgery	7 (5-10)	. (9-12)	8 (7-14)	5 (4-6)	

Po = patients operated.
[1] Median (hinges).
[2] Between not transfused patients and patients transfused with allogeneic units, after exclusions of deaths and reinterventions.
[3] Performed on ln values.
. = not calculated due to the small number of patients or records.

Note: *significant differences are shown in bold italics.*

IV.2. *Preoperative transfusion*

Twelve patients (1%) aged 75 (60 to 80) years (median, range) were transfused before surgery in 10 hospitals. The age of 10 of them fell above the upper half of the overall age distribution. The Hct value before transfusion was available in only four patients and ranged from 21 to 29%. The Hct after transfusion but before surgery (available in five patients) ranged from 28 to 45%.

IV.3. *Postoperative transfusion*

Twenty-four patients (2%) aged 76 years (median value, range 52 to 85) were transfused with red units; two of them were reoperated for bleeding. Hct values (available in approximately half of the patients) ranged from 23 to 33% (median 27%) before transfusion, and from 28 to 43% (median 33%) after transfusion of a median of two units.

V. Some in-hospital outcome variables

Table 2.4 describes some outcome variables. After surgery, an Hct value was recorded in 58% of operated patients (about one third less than had a preoperative value recorded) (Part I, Figure 0.16). The last available Hct was recorded at a median number of one day (hinges: 1-3) and showed a median value of 36% (hinges: 33-40%).

The fall between last and preoperative Hct value was $-6.6\% \pm 5.5$ in patients transfused with a mean of 2.8 ± 2.3 allogeneic red units, and $-5.1\% \pm 4.4$ in untransfused patients; in operated patients the Hct fall was $-5.5\% \pm 4.7$ with 0.4 ± 1.4 red units transfused (means $\pm$ SD). Among hospitals, the fall ranged from $-3.5\% \pm 5.9$ to $-8.0\% \pm 4.7$ (Figure 2.9), after transfusion of 0.6 ± 2.1 and 0.6 ± 0.9 red units, respectively.

Figure 2.10 shows, by hospital, the distribution of patients transfused with red units according to the last available Hct value. It is seen that about half of patients transfused showed an Hct value exceeding 33% in nearly all hospitals.

Complications of surgery

Reoperated patients were 10 years older than overall patient set, showed a median preoperative Hct value close to the lower quartile of the distribution in the overall patient set, while the median perioperative blood loss and postintervention LOS fell above the upper quartile of the distribution (Table 2.5). No information was available on the patient who died.

Median LOS before surgery was two days (hinges: 1-6) and after surgery five days (hinges: 4-7). Preoperative LOS was shorter in hospitals of central-northern Europe than in hospitals of the Mediterranean area, namely two (hinges: 1-3) versus six (hinges: 2-11) median days. A similar trend was observed also for postsurgical LOS (Figure 2.11).

69

Table 2.4. TURP: outcome variables

	EA*	DB*	IE*	EB	EC	IL	PA*	ID	PB	DKA	GBD	BA	NLB	FC	GBF	GBE	GBG	NLA	BC	GBB	FB	BB*	DKC	DKB	IA*	DA
Last Hct																										
% Po with	100	100	100	22	19	55	23	96	27	36	50	91	100	33	81	89	37	38	30	54	46	83	68	77	94	91
%, median value	38	45	45	35	33	35	41	35	38	32	38	37	39	34	38	38	36	37	35	40	34	35	35	34	37	35
range	32-43	31-48	31-48	27-44	24-45	27-47	33-43	27-45	24-47	26-45	26-44	25-47	31-47	28-46	27-46	27-53	23-48	29-48	29-46	33-49	25-45	29-39	28-44	17-44	27-46	25-44
Reoperation																										
% Po						1.6							4.0		1.9	3.0		2.6		5.7	1.0			1.6		
Mortality																										
% Po														1.8												
LOS, days																										
median	13	23	11	7	12	21	18	18	18	5	5	7	7	8	4	6	7	8	5	6	7	6	9	6	12	17
range	8-18	11-43	6-31	5-54	4-51	12-35	5-47	5-47	7-40	2-18	3-13	4-31	4-16	2-24	3-19	4-26	4-19	4-26	3-44	3-15	2-25	4-35	2-61	2-26	6-38	6-75

Po = patients operated.
No complications of transfusion were reported.
Hospital code and * = less than 20 patients.

Table 2.5. TURP: complications of surgery

	Hospital number	Patient number	Preoperative Hct, %	Age, years	Perioperative blood loss, L	Postoperative bleeding, L	Red units per patient	Last Hct %	Postoperative LOS days	Death: days after surgery
Reoperation for bleeding	11	11	39 (33-45)	81 (54-90)	• (0.4-1.3)	1.15	3 (1-11)	34 (28-40)	7 (3-50)	
recorded in	8/26	11/1 190	11/11		3/11	1/11	8/11	4/8		
deaths	1	1	30	65	0	0	0	0		5
recorded in	1/26	1/1 190								

' Median (range).
• = not calculated due to the small sample size.

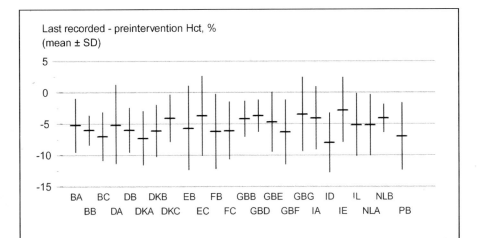

Fig 2.9. - TURP: fall of hematocrit value in operated patients. Only hospitals are reported where Hct values were recorded in at least six patients

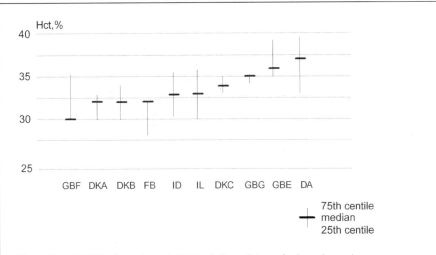

Fig 2.10. - TURP: last recorded Hct (after all transfusions have been given) in patients transfused with red units. Values are reported when available in at least six patients

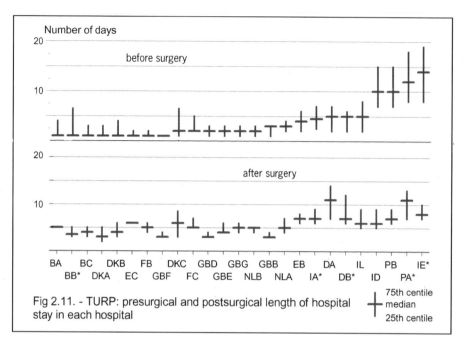

Fig 2.11. - TURP: presurgical and postsurgical length of hospital stay in each hospital

75th centile
median
25th centile

VI. Costs

Overall estimated costs of products used per operated patient accounted for ECU 34 and that of preoperative request for ECU 7.3. Costs for products used ranged from ECU 0 to 94 according to the hospital (Figure 2.12) and those for preoperative request from ECU 0 to 10. In all hospitals, the major cost was due to red unit use.

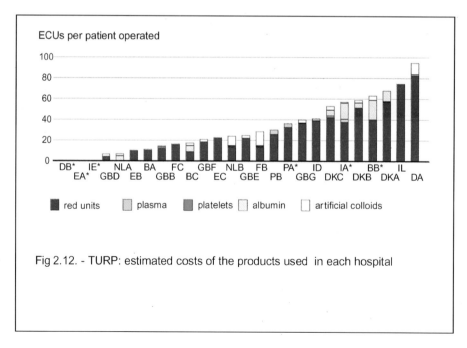

Fig 2.12. - TURP: estimated costs of the products used in each hospital

Table 2.6 summarizes the main findings in TURP.

Table 2.6. TURP: summary of main findings

			in hospitals (of 26)
Preoperative request			
percentage of operated patients with		73 (0-100)	24
MSBOS			10
T&S			17
Red units			
percentage of patients transfused			
	total	16.5 (0-46)	22
	allogeneic	15.4 (0-34)	
	autologous	0.8 (0-15)	4
	allogeneic and autologous	0.3 (0-8)	
factors implied:	transfused vs. untransfused patients		
age, years (median)		75 vs. 70	
preoperative Hct, % (median)		40 vs. 43	
perioperative blood loss, mL (median)		800 vs. 400	
reinterventions (% patients)		4.3 vs. 0.3	
deaths (% patients)		0 vs. 0.1	
last Hct, % (median)		33 vs. 38	
fall in Hct value in operated patients (last — preoperative Hct), % mean ± SD		-5.5 ± 4.7	
whole blood use (percentage of red units used as whole blood)		3 (0-37)	5
Plasma			
percentage of patients transfused		1 (0-15)	11
Albumin			
percentage of patients receiving		3 (0-19)	10
Artificial colloids			
percentage of patients receiving		20 (0-89)	16
percentage of colloids used as			
gelatin		78 (0-100)	13
dextran		12 (0-100)	4
HES		10 (0-100)	4
Other variables			
administration of anticoagulants (% patients)		34 (0-100)	23
before		15 (0-100)	19
after		14 (0-100)	12
before and after surgery		5 (0-82)	7
LOS, median day number			
before surgery		2 (1-14)	
after surgery		5 (3-11)	

In parentheses the lowest-highest value observed among hospitals.

VII. Comments on TURP

Many of the comments on CHOLE apply also to TURP. In TURP, as in CHOLE, the main demand on transfusion resources was preoperative request. This involved 73% of operated patients and was much higher than the proportion of patients receiving any product (20% for artificial colloids, 16% for red units, 3% for albumin).

Here too, preoperative assessment overestimated the probability of patients needing transfusion and did not appear to take much account of the presence of patient risk factors. Overall, four times more patients had preoperative requests than were transfused. Preoperative requesting was routine in many hospitals and patient ages and preoperative Hct were similar in patients for whom a request was and was not performed. The infrequent use of MSBOS and T&S procedure also suggests limited attention to avoiding unnecessary costs of transfusion practice.

Although blood loss in TURP is usually higher and more unpredictable than in CHOLE, closer identification of those patients most likely to need transfusion, together with the proximity of an active transfusion service, should avoid the need for routine preoperative requests.

On a large patient sample of broad origin, the probability of an operated patient being transfused with red units was 16% (compared with the 73% who had preoperative requests); however, there was a wide variability among hospitals (0-46%). Transfusion was given to older patients with lower preoperative Hct values and higher blood loss volumes. Apart from age, these factors were documented also in the clinical record, in part of the patients. Transfusion in many patients resulted in Hct values higher than generally considered necessary, [11, 12] suggesting that these are believed by clinicians to be necessary, at least in elderly patients. The last recorded Hct value of half of the patients transfused in three hospitals (GBG, GBE, DA) was 35% or higher, suggesting that a substantial number of transfusions could have safely been avoided.

A small number of patients were transfused with autologous units in four hospitals. Their younger age, likely to be associated with less comorbidity, may have suggested that they were suitable candidates for autotransfusion. In other hospitals, they might well have been candidates for no transfusion.

The use of whole blood was virtually restricted to two hospitals in Great Britain (GBE, GBF) that also used whole blood frequently for other surgical procedures.

A small use of plasma was observed. In one hospital (PB), it was remarkable that every patient received a single unit of liquid plasma, for unstated reasons.

There was little variability among hospitals in the use of albumin (0 to 10% operated patients), but the use of artificial colloids ranged from 0 to 89% of operated patients. The highest use of colloids was observed in FB, NLB, and DA. Nearly all the hospitals using albumin and/or artificial colloids were in central-northern Europe.

Differences among hospitals were also evident in some variables of practice, such as the anticoagulant type and its administration time, and preoperative LOS.

3.0. Right and left hemicolectomy (COLE) for colonic cancer

Carcinoma of the colon is the second most common malignancy occurring, exceeded in frequency only by lung cancer, and represents the second leading cause of cancer death. Surgical excision of primary tumour remains the cornerstone of therapy. Characteristically, it is a disease of older individuals with an approximately equal incidence in males and females. Although most procedures are standardized, none the less an evolution in the surgical management of selected patients with differing colonic diseases is occurring.

Case report forms were available from 995 patients in 28 hospitals and 10 countries: 694 (70%) in 17 hospitals in six central-northern European countries and 301 (30%) in 11 hospitals in four Mediterranean countries (Figure 3.1).

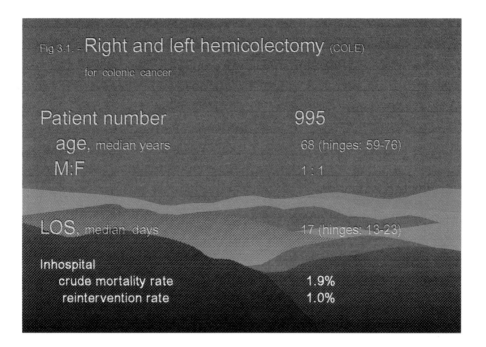

Fig 3.1 - Right and left hemicolectomy (COLE) for colonic cancer

Patient number	995
age, median years	68 (hinges: 59-76)
M:F	1 : 1
LOS, median days	17 (hinges: 13-23)
Inhospital	
crude mortality rate	1.9%
reintervention rate	1.0%

I. Patient data and some variables related to surgery

Table 3.1 reports, by hospital, the number, age and gender of patients, along with the values of some variables related to surgery.

Among hospitals, the M:F ratio was rather homogeneous and the median age ranged from 64 to 75 years. In about half of the hospitals the median age was 65 to 70 years.

The preoperative Hct value was available in 90% of patients. The median value was 38% (hinges: 34-42%). In more than two thirds of the hospitals the median preoperative Hct was 37% or higher and in the remaining third it was 34 to 36%.

Table 3.1. COLE: patient data and some variables related to surgery

	PA	EB*	GRC	ID	DKA	IE*	IL	ED*	EA	GBG	PB*	FD	FA	GBD	FC	DKB	GBE	NLB	DA	DKC*	FB*	NLA	BC	EC	BB	IA	BA	DB
Patient number	22	14	27	44	46	8	21	11	50	30	14	57	36	42	45	52	54	39	31	12	14	36	50	54	59	36	59	32
Age median years	65	72	68	67	68	69	68	63	69	72	66	67	69	72	66	72	75	71	64	74	70	65	66	70	65	75	65	65
range	45-81	57-80	42-87	37-91	20-91	55-82	18-85	44-85	42-91	41-86	32-79	26-91	36-87	41-87	29-90	26-89	46-91	30-88	24-82	56-87	20-90	42-84	36-90	33-91	24-88	35-88	20-84	46-81
M:F ratio	0.7	6.0	0.9	0.7	1.3	0.3	0.9	2.7	1.0	1.1	0.7	1.2	0.9	0.8	1.4	0.6	1.1	0.8	0.9	0.5	0.5	1.4	0.8	1.8	0.9	1.1	1.1	0.6
Preoperative Hct % Po with	95	86	100	89	72	87	71	100	90	87	100	88	86	90	93	88	96	100	97	92	100	100	98	85	97	89	100	100
%, median	37	37	41	38		39	34	39	35	35	35	38	41	37	39	36	36	40	38	36	38	40	37	40	39	34	37	38
range	27-45	28-46	28-48	26-50	30-49	30-40	24-47	33-46	13-48	18-46	25-48	27-49	26-50	26-50	26-50	27-47	17-50	32-47	24-46	24-44	26-43	27-50	13-48	22-48	24-49	27-45	27-49	29-53
Drugs[1] Recipients % Po	41	64	96	11	22	12	95	57	98	17	57	98	64	90	95	13	91	100	93	92	100	100	28	92	30	30	98	97
Anaesthesia regional or combined % Po	21	21	4			9			2					14			26	20		33	100	42	58		10	3	3	87
Duration of surgery % Po with	63	100	59	2	89	100		100	100	57	100			83		94	61	77		100	64	89	80	100	78	33	73	
median minutes	155	187	135	•	140	116		110	170	90	185			135		100	105	117		102	150	150	155	180	175	207	185	
range	150-190	105-300	45-215		60-270	90-130		60-180	80-200	60-200	60-240			55-300		50-170	50-205	60-190		60-165	90-240	90-225	60-270	90-225	120-330	120-330	120-405	
Blood loss perioperative % Po with	4				76	50		82	74	30			19	57	75	88	18	95	74	100	7	94	90	20	75	8		100
median L	•				0.30	0.40		0.40	0.40	0.50			0.80	0.45	0.13	0.30	0.40	0.30	0.40	0.32	•	0.50	0.45	0.35	0.50	•		0.80
range					0.1-1.1	0.2-0.5		0.2-1.2	0.1-1.5				0.1-0.8	0.1-1.2	0.0-0.5	0.1-5.5	0.2-1.4	0.1-2.0	0.1-1.5	0.0-2.0		0.0-2.0	0.0-2.2	0.1-2.2	0.0-4.0			0.1-4.5
postoperative % Po with	•			13					6				92	36	78		29	13			93	19	88	65	95	8	83	
median L				•					•				0.27	0.30	0.08		0.19	•			0.69	0.15	0.32	0.26	0.26	•	0.24	
range													0.0-0.8	0.0-1.7	0.0-1.0		0.0-3.3				0.0-2.2	0.1-0.4	0.0-4.7	0.0-1.2	0.0-1.8		0.0-1.7	

Po = patients operated.
[1] only anticoagulants were administered.
Hospital code and * = less than 20 patients.
• = not calculated due to the small sample size.

Of operated patients, 67% received a drug acting on the coagulation system: 39% only after surgery, 15% both before and after surgery, 12% only before surgery, and 1% intraoperatively. Before surgery, low-dose heparin (23%) and aspirin/NSAID (4%) were used, and after surgery, low-dose heparin (54%). Most hospitals used anticoagulants mainly after surgery, a few mainly before surgery or both before and after surgery (Figure 3.2).

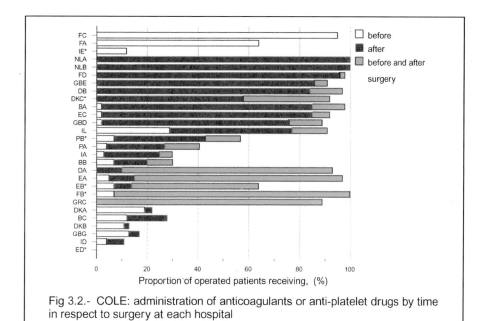

Fig 3.2.- COLE: administration of anticoagulants or anti-platelet drugs by time in respect to surgery at each hospital

Anaesthesia was general in 88%, regional in 1% and combined in 11% of patients. In two hospitals (DB, BC) regional or combined anaesthesia was used for most patients.

Information on duration of surgery was available in 58% of patients. The median time was 150 minutes (hinges: 115-180) and varied among hospitals by a factor of more than two.

Blood loss data were available in 62% of patients; perioperatively in 30%, postoperatively in 16%, and both peri- and postoperatively in 16%. Data were more often available in hospitals of central-northern Europe. The median value was 0.4 L (hinges: 0.2-0.7) perioperatively, and 0.2 L (hinges: 0.1-0.5) postoperatively. According to reported perioperative blood loss, 4.1% patients bled more than 1.5 L (Figure 3.3).

II. Transfusion data

Table 3.2 shows, by hospital, the percentage of patients receiving each product and the amount of product administered to recipients. Differences among hospitals in the products used were

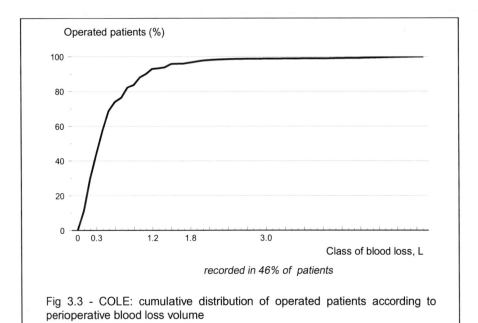

Fig 3.3 - COLE: cumulative distribution of operated patients according to perioperative blood loss volume

less remarkable than in other interventions, indicating a more homogenous approach to the procedure. Exceptions are given by some hospitals (PA, EB, GRC), where only blood components were used. In hospitals located in four of the 10 countries (Belgium, France, the Netherlands, Germany) the same kind of products were used.

II.1.0. *Red units*

In all 406 (41%) patients received 1 216 red units in 27 of 28 hospitals. The percentage of patients transfused differed widely among hospitals, i.e. from 0 to 78%. In hospitals of central-northern European countries it was slightly lower than in those of the Mediterranean area (RR = 0.8 (0.6 to 0.9)). In transfused patients the median number of units was two (hinges: 2-4), ranging from one to four among hospitals. Of operated patients, 5.9% received a number of units higher than four (Figure 3.4).

II.1.1. *Autologous transfusion*

In eight hospitals, 44 autologous red units were transfused to 24 patients (2%): 40 PABD units to 21 patients and four PIH units (FB) to three patients.

II.1.2. *Whole blood*

7% of allogeneic red units were used as whole blood; three hospitals accounting for 5.6% (BA, GBE, GRC). There, the proportion of whole blood represented 39, 25 and 17%, respectively, of the red units used.

78

Table 3.2. COLE: transfusion data

	PA	EB*	GRC	ID	DKA	IE*	IL	ED*	EA	GBG	PB*	FD	FA	GBD	FC	DKB	GBE	NLB	DA	DKC*	FB*	NLA	BC	EC	BB	IA	BA	DB
[1] (autotransfusion)		-				-		-			-									-	-					-		-
Red units																												
patients transfused/operated (%)	27.3	78.6	77.8	34.1	36.9		47.6	54.5	36.0	50.0	57.1	7.0	16.7	21.4	22.2	32.7	38.9	41.0	38.7	50.0	50.0	41.7	50.0	53.7	47.4	58.3	54.2	68.7
units per transfused patient — median	1	•	4	2	2		2		2	2		3	2	3	3	2	2	2	2			2.5	2	2	2	2	2	2
hinges	1-1	•	2-4	2-3	1-3		1-4		2-3	2-2		2-5	2-3	2-3	3-4	2-3	2-4	2-4	2-2.5			2-4	1-3	2-4	2-3	2-3	1-4	2-4
Plasma																												
patients transfused/operated (%)	22.7	21.4	14.8	6.8		37.5					57.1	1.7		2.4	6.7	1.9			9.7		14.3	19.4	32.0	13.0	10.2		37.3	28.1
units per transfused patient — median	2	•	6.5	•		•					•	•		•	•	•			•		•	4	4	3	3		4	2
hinges	2-2	•	1-12	•		•					•	•		•	•	•			•		•	2-4	4-9	2-8	2-4		2-6	2-2
Platelets																												
patients transfused/operated (%)	4.5															1.9												
Albumin																												
patients administered/operated (%)	11.4				28.3	12.5	23.8	9.1				15.8	7.1		2.2	46.1	1.8	5.1	19.3	25.0	57.1	63.9	98.0	1.8	91.5	86.1	89.8	37.5
grams per recipient — median	11				13	•	nos	•				21	51		•	23	•	•	60	•	•	21	126	•	83	42	101	26
hinges	11-22				13-41							21-21	33-103			13-36			42-78			21-41	104-166		61-125	31-96	61-121	13-26
Lyophilized plasma																												
patients transfused/operated (%)								9.1															2					
Colloids																												
patients administered/operated (%)									24.0	50.0	7.1	71.9	36.1	54.8	33.3	53.8	57.4	66.7	58.1	41.7	42.9	63.9	80.0	1.8	30.5	2.8	13.5	93.7
litres per recipient — median									0.5	0.5		0.5	0.5	1.0	0.5	0.5	0.5	0.5	0.7			0.5	0.5	•	1.0	•	0.5	0.5
hinges									0.5-0.5	0.5-0.5		0.5-1.0	0.5-1.0	0.5-1.5	0.5-0.5	0.5-1.0	0.5-1.0	0.5-1.0	0.5-1.0			0.5-1.0	0.5-1.0		0.5-2.5		0.5-1.2	0.5-1.0
Patients for whom red units transfused were not recorded (percent operated)																						2.8						

Hospitals are aggregated according to the products used.

Hospital code and * = less than 20 patients.

• = not calculated due to the small sample size.

nos = not otherwise specified.

[1] autotransfusion use.

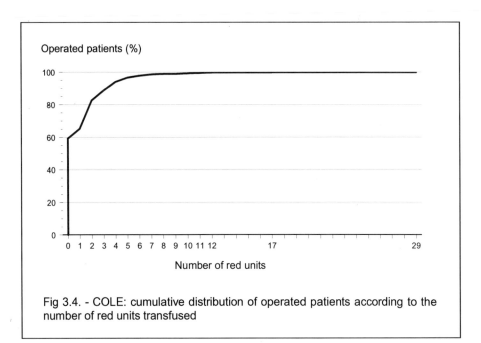

Fig 3.4. - COLE: cumulative distribution of operated patients according to the number of red units transfused

II.1.3. *Time of transfusion*

Transfusion episodes during LOS were more widespread than in the other studied surgical procedures (Figure 3.5). The mean number of transfusion episodes per patient transfused was 1.4.

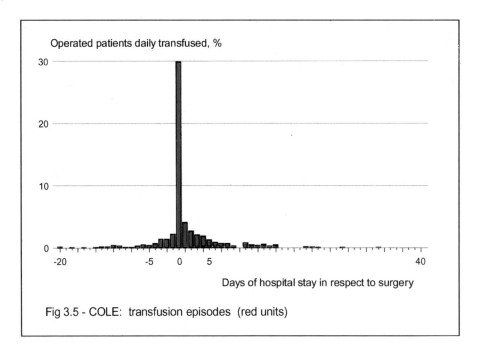

Fig 3.5 - COLE: transfusion episodes (red units)

The proportion of patients transfused only postoperatively (Figure 3.6) was large in two hospitals (FA, FD). In both these hospitals the overall percentage of operated patients who were transfused was the lowest observed among hospitals.

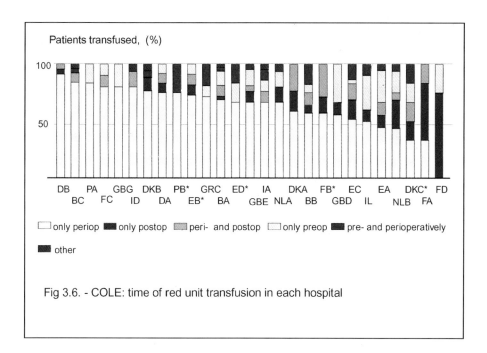

Fig 3.6. - COLE: time of red unit transfusion in each hospital

II.2.0. *Plasma*

In all 366 units of plasma were transfused to 104 patients (10%) in two thirds of the hospitals. In transfused patients the median number of units was four (hinges: 2-6). Plasma was used in all hospitals of Belgium, Germany and Portugal (Figure 3.7); however, Belgian hospitals (providing 17% of the COLE patients) accounted for 42% of all plasma recipients and 38% of the units transfused. As a consequence, the percentage of plasma recipients in hospitals of central-northern Europe was one and a half that of the Mediterranean area (RR = 1.5 (1 to 3)).

Thirty patients received plasma as unique blood component and the remaining 74 patients along with red units, 13 of them within 24 hours.

Of 366 units of plasma, 11 (3%) were autologous (hospital DB), 164 (45%) fresh frozen, 119 (32%) from apheresis (hospitals BA, BC) and 72 (20%) liquid (hospitals EC, NLA, PB).

II.3.0. *Albumin*

In all 25 977 g of albumin were administered to 314 patients (32%) in about three quarters of the hospitals. In recipients, the median amount was 62 g (hinges: 21-109) and ranged among hospitals from 11 to 126 g. The percentage of patients administered with albumin in hospitals of

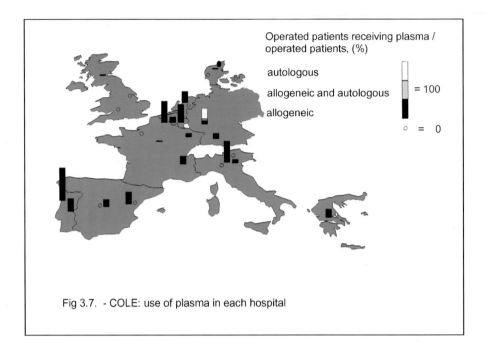

Fig 3.7. - COLE: use of plasma in each hospital

central-northern Europe was twice (Figure 3.8) that of the Mediterranean area (RR = 2 (2 to 3)). In fact, 50% of albumin recipients and 70% of all albumin used was observed in Belgian hospitals.

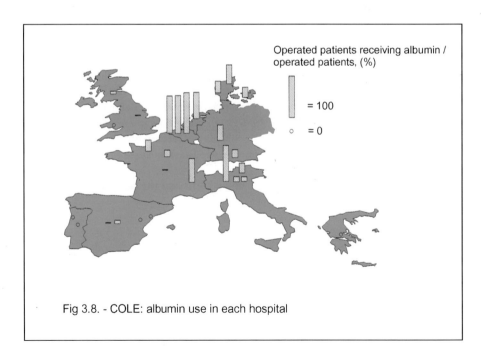

Fig 3.8. - COLE: albumin use in each hospital

II.4.0. *Artificial colloids*

In all 275 L of artificial colloids were administered in approximately three quarters of the hospitals to 355 patients (36%). About one third of recipients were in three hospitals (BC, FD, DB). The percentage of patients administered with colloids in hospitals of central-northern Europe was eight times (Figure 3.9) that of hospitals in the Mediterranean area (RR = 8 (6 to 12)). The median volume administered to recipients was 0.5 L (hinges: 0.5-1.0).

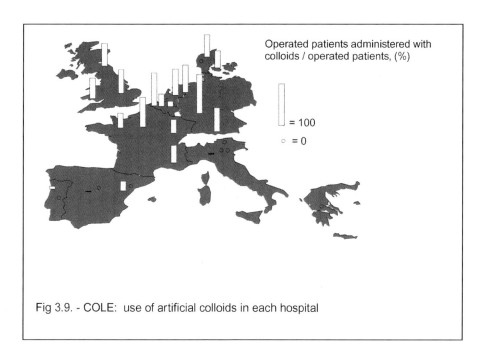

Fig 3.9. - COLE: use of artificial colloids in each hospital

Gelatin was used in eight of the 20 hospitals, dextran in three, HES in one and in those remaining a combination of colloids (Figure 3.10). In recipients, the median volume of artificial colloids varied among hospitals according to the type of colloid: from 0.5 to 1.5 L for gelatin, from 0.5 to 2.5 L for dextran and from 0.5 to 1.0 L for HES.

The variety in the clinical use of the studied products among hospitals is shown in Figure 3.11 and among hospitals aggregated according to the country in Figure 3.12.

III. Reasons for transfusion documented in the medical record

III.1. *Red units*

A reason was documented in 25% of recipients (Figure 3.13). Hospitals documenting were mainly of central-northern Europe. The value of Hct and the presence of bleeding were the more frequently stated reasons.

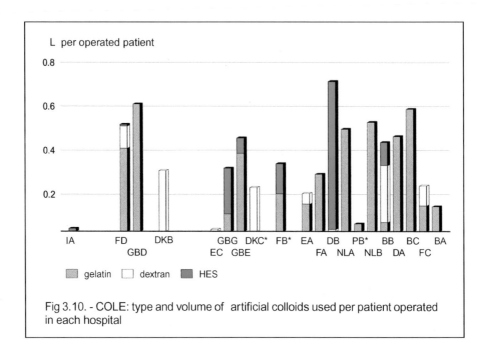

Fig 3.10. - COLE: type and volume of artificial colloids used per patient operated in each hospital

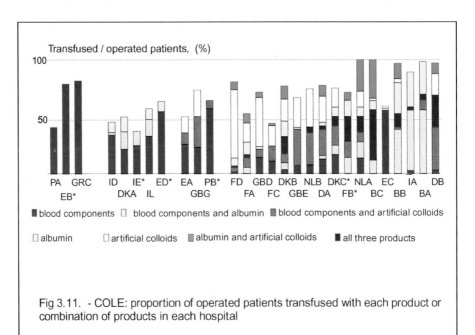

Fig 3.11. - COLE: proportion of operated patients transfused with each product or combination of products in each hospital

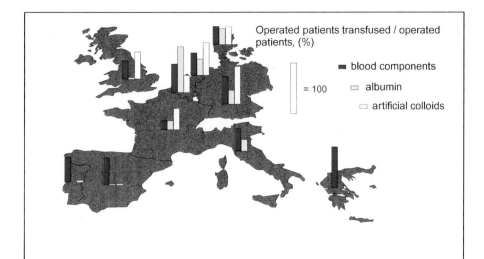

Fig 3.12. - COLE: use of the products in hospitals aggregated by country

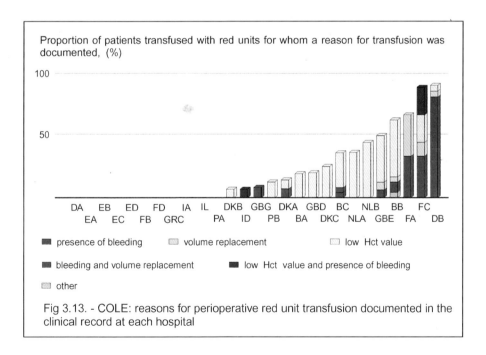

Fig 3.13. - COLE: reasons for perioperative red unit transfusion documented in the clinical record at each hospital

III.2. *Plasma*

Reasons were found in 38% of patients from five hospitals, all of them of central-northern Europe. A PT value of 52% (39 to 68%), median (range) was recorded in 27% of the recipients; volume replacement, bleeding or both in 11%.

III.3. *Albumin*

Reasons were found in 12% of patients from eight hospitals. Volume replacement was reported for nearly all patients.

III.4. *Artificial colloids*

Reasons were found in 22% of the recipients from five hospitals, mainly represented by volume replacement.

IV. Variables associated with red unit transfusion

IV.1. *Transfused versus untransfused patients*

The profile of patients transfused and not transfused with red units during the hospital stay is reported in Table 3.3. A higher age and blood loss, and a lower preoperative Hct value characterized the sub-set of patients transfused, even after exclusion of reinterventions and deaths.

The few patients transfused with autologous red units were younger than other patient sub-groups and underwent surgery with preoperative Hct values lower than untransfused patients; the latter was likely due to the withdrawal of PABD units.

IV.2. *Preoperative transfusion*

In all 72 patients (7%) were transfused with red units before surgery in 23 of 28 hospitals. Their median age and M:F ratio were similar to those of untransfused patients (Table 3.4). Before surgery, their Hct was raised to 32% ±6.0 which was still lower than that of patients who received no preoperative transfusion. The preoperative LOS of the transfused patients was nearly twice that of untransfused patients.

IV.3. *Perioperative patient transfusion*

Indicator: proportion of operated patients perioperatively transfused with red units (mean percent-age ± SE)
Hospitals: 19 (86%) of 22 enrolling 20 or more patients
Patients: 786 (81%) of 969, after exclusion of deaths and reinterventions
Variables: age, gender, preintervention Hct, blood loss

On average, the probability of a patient being transfused (Part I, Figure 0.14) was higher in females than in males (+8%), after adjustment for age, and also in patients aged over 73 years

Table 3.3. COLE: profiles of patients transfused and not transfused with red units during the hospital stay

	Patients transfused			Patients not transfused	95% confidence interval of the difference[2]
	allogeneic	allogeneic and autologous	autologous		
Patient number	382	5	19	589	
Age, years[1]	*70 (60-78)*	69 (65-75)	68 (52-78)	*67 (58-76)*	*−1.2 to −4.8*
M:F	0.94	0.67	0.58	1.0	3 to 10
Hct[1] preoperative, %	*36 (31-39)*	37(37-40)	35(31-38)	*40(36-43)*	*3.7 to 5.1*
Percentage of patients with	92	100	100	91	
Anaesthesia, regional and/or combined,% Po	13	80	31	10	
Anticoagulants, % Po	64	100	84	68	
Duration of surgery,[1] minutes	160 (120-190)	240 (240-240)	165 (150-185)	150 (104-180)	
Percentage of patients with	66	20	32	54	
Blood loss,[1] L perioperative	*0.47 (0.3-1.0)*	.	.	*0.3 (0.2-0.5)*	*0.7 to 0.5*[3]
Percentage of patients with	48			44	
total	1.0 (0.5-1.5)			0.5 (0.3-0.9)	
Percentage of patients with	19			17	
Percentage of patients transfused with					
plasma	17.0	100	21.0		
albumin	40.0	40	10.5	26.7	
artificial colloids	34.8	80	52.6	35.4	
PABD, % patients		100	100		
Stated reason for transfusion, % Pt	24	80	47		
Reintervention for bleeding, % Po	2.1	20		0.17	
In-hospital crude mortality rate, % Po	3.14		10.5	0.85	
Last Hct (%)[1]	34 (32-38)	33 (30-38)	36 (31-39)	34 (31-37)	
Percentage of patients with	94	100	100	87	
Hospital stay, day number[1]	19 (15-28)	17 (14-25)	13 (12-21)	15 (12-21)	
before surgery	6 (2-10)	1 (1-4)	2 (1-6)	3 (2-7)	
after surgery	13 (10-16)	13 (10-13)	11 (9-12)	11 (9-140)	

[1] Median (hinges).
[2] Between patients not transfused and patients transfused with allogeneic units, after exclusion of deaths and reinterventions.
[3] Performed on ln values.
Po = patients operated.
Pt = patients transfused.
· = not calculated due to the small number of patients or records.
Note: *significant differences are shown in bold italics.*

(difference between the highest and lowest age class = +8%), after adjustment for gender. As might be expected, the higher the blood loss volume the higher the probability of transfusion (difference between the highest and lowest class of blood loss = +25%), and the higher the preoperative Hct value the lower the probability of transfusion (difference between the highest and lowest class of Hct = −35%), after adjustment for age and gender.

Age affected patient transfusion in nine of 19 hospitals (but in two hospitals older patients had a lower probability of being transfused); gender in 13 of 19 hospitals (but in three hospitals males were transfused more than females), preoperative Hct in nine of 13 hospitals (Figure 3.14) and blood loss in three of seven hospitals (Figure 3.15) when extremes of the classes are considered.

Table 3.4. COLE: some characteristics of patients transfused and not transfused with red units before surgery

	Patients transfused	Patients not transfused	95% confidence interval of the difference
Patient number	72	923	
Age, years[1]	68 ± 15	66 ± 13	−5.2 to 1.2
Percentage of males	47	50	−9 to 15
Hct, %[1]			
pretransfusion	27 ± 3		
percentage of patients with	37		
postransfusion	33 ± 5		
percentage of patients with	46		
before surgery, %[1]	*32 ± 6.0*	*38 ± 5.0*	*4.8 to 7.2*
percentage of patients with	98	92	
Units per patient transfused[1]	2.5 ± 1.0		
Preoperative LOS, days[1]	10 ± 7	6 ± 8	

[1] Means ± SD.

Note: **significant differences are shown in bold italics.**

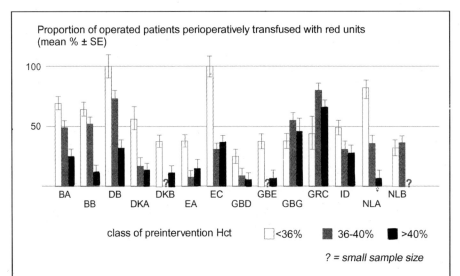

Fig 3.14. - COLE: effect of preoperative Hct on the proportion of patients perioperatively transfused with red units in each hospital, after adjustment for age and gender. Also hospitals are reported where the size of a Hct class was small

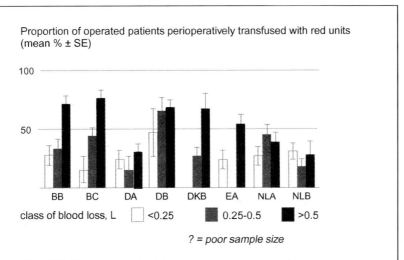

Fig 3.15. - COLE: effect of blood loss on the proportion of patients perioperatively transfused with red units in each hospital, after adjustment for age and gender. Also hospitals are reported where the size of a blood loss class was small

The qualitative effect of these variables in the individual hospitals is summarized in Figure 3.16. There were some hospitals, such as DKB, where most of the predisposing factors affected the probability of a patient being transfused in an understandable way. In contrast, there were hospitals where a rationale based on the variables under study could not be discerned (DA). In other hospitals, the recorded data were insufficient to permit this form of analysis.

The probability of a patient being transfused varied with the hospital, even after adjustment for age, gender and preoperative Hct (Figure 3.17): from $14\% \pm 4.4$ to $72\% \pm 5.3$ (difference between the highest and lowest value = 58%), and even further adjustment for blood loss (Figure 3.18) from $27\% \pm 6.8$ to $70\% \pm 10.7$ (difference between the highest and lowest value = 43%).

In ascending order, differences in the proportion of patients transfused attributable to age were 8%, to gender 8%, to blood loss 25%, to preoperative Hct 35% and to other, unknown variables associated with the hospital 43%.

IV.4. *Postoperative transfusion*

Table 3.5 shows the profiles of patients transfused in the postoperative period compared with those who did not receive postoperative transfusion. After exclusion of deaths and reoperations, only a high postoperative blood loss characterized patients transfused. The Hct value resulting after transfusion was similar to that of untransfused patients. The 'trigger' or threshold Hct value for postoperative red unit transfusion was rather consistent (28% ± 3.7 among the 61 patients). More than two thirds of patients postoperatively transfused were from particular hospitals (BA, BB, DKA, EC, NLB).

	age, years >73 vs <63	gender F vs M	presurgery Hct, % >40 vs <36	blood loss, L >0.5 vs 0.25
BA	↑		↓	/
BB		↑	↓	↑
BC	↑	↑	?	↑
DA			?	
DB			↓	
DKA	↓	↓	↓	?
DKB	↑	↑	↓	?
EA	↑			↑
EC	↑	↑	↓	/
FC		↑	?	?
GBD				?
GBE	?		↓	/
GBG		↓		/
GRC		↑		/
IA	↓	↑	?	/
ID	↑	↑	↓	/
IL	↑	↑	?	/
NLA		↑	↓	
NLB		↓	?	

↑ increase   ↓ decrease   blank = no variation

/ = data not available   ? = poor sample size

Fig 3.16. - COLE: variables affecting the proportion of patients perioperatively transfused with red units in each hospital. The comparison is performed between the highest and lowest class of each variable

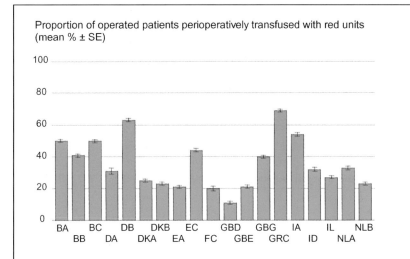

Proportion of operated patients perioperatively transfused with red units (mean % ± SE)

Fig 3.17. - COLE: probability of a patient being perioperatively transfused with red units in each hospital after adjustment for age, gender and preoperative Hct

Table 3.5. COLE: some characteristics of patients transfused and not transfused with red units in the postoperative period,[1] after exclusion of deaths and reinterventions

	Patients transfused	Patients not transfused	95% confidence interval of the difference
Patient number	61	908	
Age, years[2]	69 ± 15	66 ± 14	−6.6 to 0.6
Percentage of males	46	50	−8 to 15
Hct, pretransfusion %[2]	28 ± 3.7		
percentage of patients with	64		
Postoperative blood loss, mL[2]	*5.9 ± 1.1*	*5.3 ± 1.4*	*0.32 to 0.94[3]*
percentage of patients with	46	31	
Units per patient transfused[2]	2.8 ± 16		
Last Hct, %[2]	35 ± 5.4	35 ± 4.9	−0.7 to 2.5
percentage of patients with	62	90	
Postsurgical LOS, days[2]	20 ± 10	12 ± 5.8	

[1] From the fourth day after surgery to discharge.
[2] Mean ± SD.
[3] Performed on ln values.

Note: **significant differences are shown in bold italics.**

V. Some outcome variables

Table 3.6 describes some outcome variables. After surgery, at least one Hct value was available in 90% of operated patients and was recorded at a median of six days (hinges: 3-9) after. The median value was 34% (hinges: 31-38%). In nearly two thirds of the hospitals it was 34% or higher, and in the remaining third it was 30 to 33%.

In transfused patients, the last Hct was recorded after all transfusions were given at a median number of six days (hinges: 3-10) after surgery. The median value was 35% (hinges: 32-38%). In eight hospitals, 75% or more of transfused patients (Figure 3.19) were discharged with Hct values higher than 33%. Six of eight hospitals were from central-northern European countries.

The mean Hct fall in untransfused patients was −4.9% ± 4.8 and ranged among hospitals from −1.7% ± 7.4 to −8.5% ± 5.7. In patients transfused with a mean of 2.5 ± 1.3 red units, the fall in Hct was 0.3% ± 6.0 and ranged among hospitals from 2.0% ± 7.4 to −2.6% ± 2.9.

Complications of transfusion

A complication of allogeneic blood transfusion was reported in six patients in four hospitals: a skin reaction in one patient (BA) and fever/rigors in five patients (BA, DKB, NLA, GRC).

Table 3.6. COLE: outcome variables

	PA	EB*	GRC	ID	DKA	IE*	IL	ED*	EA	GBG	PB*	FD	FA	GBD	FC	DKB	GBE	NLB	DA	DKC*	FB*	NLA	BC	EC	BB	IA	BA	DB
Last Hct																												
% Po with	91	100	93	95	93	62	100	100	80	87	86	63	97	97	95	96	79	92	100	100	100	42	100	89	97	100	100	100
%, median	35	35	40	33	36	34	34	37	30	35	31	33	33	33	36	31	33	37	33	35	35	33	35	36	35	33	36	34
range	27-47	23-48	29-50	26-47	27-43	33-38	27-45	29-42	22-44	28-43	27-38	23-44	23-40	23-44	27-50	23-47	19-56	27-44	24-41	31-44	29-39	23-41	29-50	26-47	25-47	25-44	28-46	26-41
Complications of transfusion																												
allogeneic, % Pt			9.1										5.5			5.9						5.5						
autologous, % Pt																											4.8	
Reoperation																												
% Po					6.5											1.9	1.8	2.5					2.0					3.1
Mortality																												
% Po					4.3				6.0			1.7		2.4		1.9	1.8	7.7		16.6		2.8	4.0		3.4			
LOS																												
median, days	19	26	19	20	24	31	19	28	20	14	26	13	16	13	15	13	12	16	18	19	18	15	17	23	16	17	18	13
range	11-41	10-62	7-38	9-54	12-56	17-41	13-47	10-43	10-74	8-31	13-46	7-53	8-49	8-33	9-46	2-59	8-23	12-48	9-171	7-47	11-33	10-30	11-47	9-51	10-55	9-46	10-50	8-35

Po = patients operated.
Pt = patients transfused.
Hospital code and * = less than 20 patients.

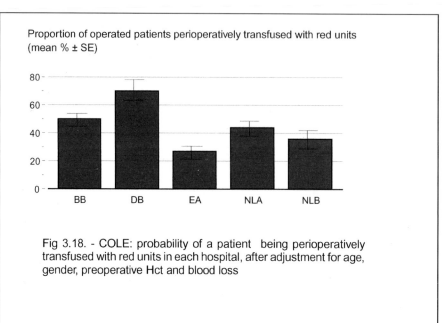

Proportion of operated patients perioperatively transfused with red units
(mean % ± SE)

Fig 3.18. - COLE: probability of a patient being perioperatively
transfused with red units in each hospital, after adjustment for age,
gender, preoperative Hct and blood loss

Complications of surgery

Three out of 10 patients who underwent a reoperation for bleeding subsequently died. Age and
the number of red units transfused (and possibly blood loss volumes) fell above the upper
quartile of overall patient distribution. LOS after surgery was twice as long as that of the overall
group of COLE patients (Table 3.7). Three of the 19 patients who died were previously
reoperated for bleeding.

Median LOS before surgery was four days (hinges: 2-8) and after surgery 12 days (hinges: 10-
14). Preoperative LOS in hospitals of central-northern Europe was shorter than in hospitals of
the Mediterranean area, namely three (hinges: 2-6) versus seven (hinges: 4-12) median days
(Figure 3.20).

VI. Costs

Overall costs of products used were estimated at ECU 150 per operated patient. In Figure 3.21
they are shown subdivided according to the product. The costs of colloids were similar to those
of red units. Among hospitals, costs ranged from ECU 29 to 456 per operated patient (Figure
3.22). The impact of albumin use on the high costs in the Belgian hospitals is obvious.

94

Results — Individual surgical procedures

Table 3.7. COLE: complications of surgery

	Hospital number	Patient number	Age, years[1]	Gender M:F	Preoperative Hct %[1]	Perioperative blood loss, L[1]	Postoperative bleeding, L[1]	Red units per patient[1]	Last Hct %[1]	Postsurgical LOS, days[1]	Death:[1] days after surgery
Reoperation for bleeding		10	74 (49-85)	3:2	36 (33-46)	0.3 (0.1-5.5)	• (0.7-4.8)	6 (2-29)	• (32-40)	25 (1-39)	• (1-19)
recorded in	7/28	10/995			7/10	8/10	3/10	9/10	4/9		3/10
deaths		19	79 (43-91)	9:10	34 (24-47)	1.2 (0.1-5.5)	0.1 (0.2-2.8)	3 (1-29)	32 (23-40)	14 (1-53)	
recorded in	11/28	19/995			17/19	15/19	5/19	14/19	8/14		

[1] Median (range).
• = not calculated due to the small number of patients or records.

95

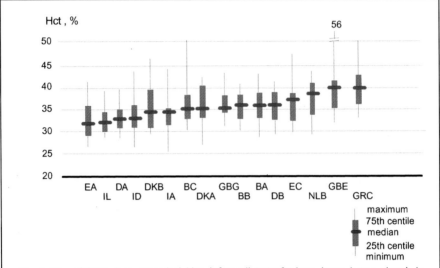

Fig 3.19. - COLE: last recorded Hct (after all transfusions have been given) in patients transfused with red units in each hospital. Each distribution refers to ten or more patients

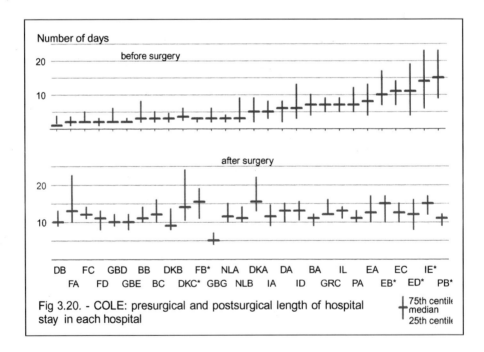

Fig 3.20. - COLE: presurgical and postsurgical length of hospital stay in each hospital

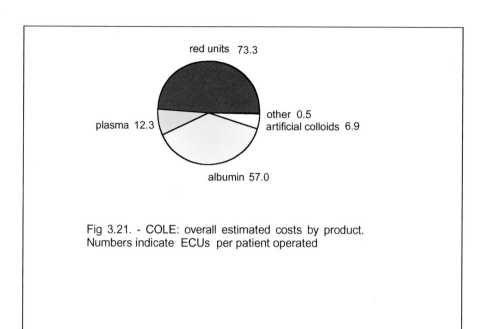

red units 73.3

plasma 12.3

other 0.5
artificial colloids 6.9

albumin 57.0

Fig 3.21. - COLE: overall estimated costs by product.
Numbers indicate ECUs per patient operated

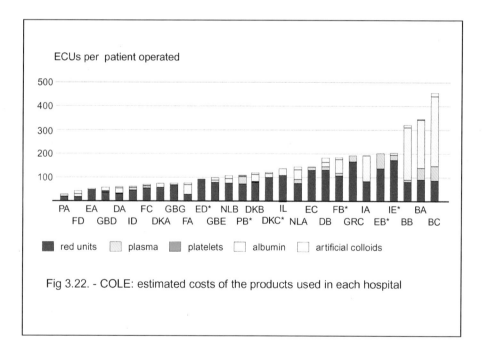

ECUs per patient operated

red units plasma platelets albumin artificial colloids

Fig 3.22. - COLE: estimated costs of the products used in each hospital

97

VII. Comments on COLE

COLE patients received red units (41% of patients operated), artificial colloids (36%), albumin (32%) and plasma (10%). These proportions, however, differed greatly among hospitals, even within a country: from 0 to 79% for red units, 0 to 94% for albumin, 0 to 98% for artificial colloids and 0 to 57% for plasma. Similar differences were also observed in the quantity of products administered to recipients: from one to four for red units, 11 to 126 g for albumin, 0.5 to 1 L for artificial colloids and two to six units for plasma. In some hospitals (BA, BB, BC, DB, NLA), the greater the range of products used, the higher was the proportion of recipients of each product as well as the amount of each product administered.

The proportion of patients who were transfused with red units differed among hospitals by a factor of more than 10. It is not known if or how some hospitals selected patients for surgery, nor whether the 'case-mix' differed among hospitals with respect to disease staging and comorbidity, in the proportions of right and left colectomies and in the specific surgical techniques used. It is likely however, that such differences would be at least partly reflected by differences in preoperative Hct values and blood loss volumes.

Some variables were found to influence the transfusion of patients with red units, notably the Hct value (pre-, peri- and postoperatively) and blood losses (peri- and postoperatively). However, the proportion of patients perioperatively transfused still differed among hospitals, even after adjustment for age, gender, preoperative Hct and blood loss, indicating that other, unidentified factors were operative. This is confirmed also by the different effect of the studied variables in some hospitals on patient transfusion. In GRC, for instance, the highest values of the last Hct were observed along with the highest proportion of patients transfused, whereas in FD the lowest values of the last Hct were observed associated with the lowest proportion of patients transfused. In the latter hospital, furthermore, perioperative transfusion was withheld and red units were administered postoperatively, presumably to reach an Hct value deemed appropriate before the patient's discharge.

Therefore, hospitals seemed to differ in their transfusion strategies. This is confirmed by the different distribution of transfused patients according to the last available Hct. In some of the hospitals, half of the transfused patients had an Hct value lower than 33%, whereas in others it was 35% or higher, indicating overtransfusion by conventional criteria.

Of patients scheduled for surgery, 7% were transfused before intervention, a finding consistent with the pathology. In these patients, the post-transfusion Hct value of $32\% \pm 6$ was apparently considered to be more appropriate for the procedure to be done than the pretransfusion value of $27\% \pm 3$. The long preoperative LOS and transfusion may have identified a more severely ill sub-set of patients.

The proportion of patients postoperatively transfused was similar to that of patients preoperatively transfused. Low Hct and high postoperative blood loss were the variables associated with postoperative transfusion. The threshold for transfusion was an Hct value of $28\% \pm 3.7$. In some hospitals the administration of long-lasting colloids may have resulted in a slight haemodilution: the resulting spurious anaemia could trigger transfusion. In the overall patient set, however, the last Hct value was similar in patients transfused and not transfused postoperatively, and the proportion of patients receiving colloids was similar in both patient groups.

Autotransfusion (almost all PABD) was infrequently used. In some hospitals, however, auto-transfusion was used in up to 25% of patients. These patients had not had sufficient time to reconstitute the red cell mass and to regain pre-donation Hct values. This made it almost certain that they would be transfused. The use of autotransfusion in COLE is usually not advised, [13-15] both because anaemia is often present due to the tumour (PABD, PIH) and possible contamination of the operative field (IBS).

It seems probable that plasma was given mainly for volume replacement, taking account of the (infrequent) stated reasons for transfusion and the frequent use of liquid plasma. This is widely considered to be an inappropriate indication for plasma transfusion. [12] In one hospital (DB) autologous plasma obtained from PABD was separated, frozen and then given back to patients, in the majority of the cases in a dose of one unit per patient. The rationale for this expensive practice is not known. In two hospitals in Belgium, apheresis plasma was also used in a percentage of operated patients and at doses much higher than in other hospitals. In the Belgian hospitals, this use of plasma was accompanied by a high use of albumin and colloids.

The large extracellular fluid losses characteristic of intra-abdominal surgical procedures such as colectomy were managed by the great majority of the hospitals (25 of 28) by giving colloids. However, great differences in the use of the various colloids were observed among hospitals, even within a country. Hospitals of central-northern Europe used three times more albumin and eight times more colloids than those of the Mediterranean area. Limited availability of these products in some countries partly explains the differences. However, variations are evident even when hospitals within one country are compared, since within a country health-care organization and the availability of products may be expected to be rather uniform. It seems probable that the same variation relates mainly to the preferences of individual clinicians (or possibly to the decision of purchasing offices).

4.0. Unilateral total hip replacement (THR) for osteoarthritis

In developed countries, hip arthroplasty for arthrosis is one of most common major elective surgical procedures that dramatically improves the quality of patient life. In those countries, candidates to THR represent an important component of the waiting list. Male to female ratio is between 1:2.5 to 1:7, modal age between 65 and 74 years, mortality rate <1%, LOS is usually 12 to 15 days. THR patients are appropriate candidates for preoperative autologous blood donation since the surgical schedule is usually anticipated and blood replacement is often needed.

Case report forms were available from 1 647 patients in 31 hospitals and 10 countries: 948 (57%) in 16 hospitals in six central-northern European countries and 699 (43%) in 15 hospitals in four Mediterranean countries (Figure 4.1).

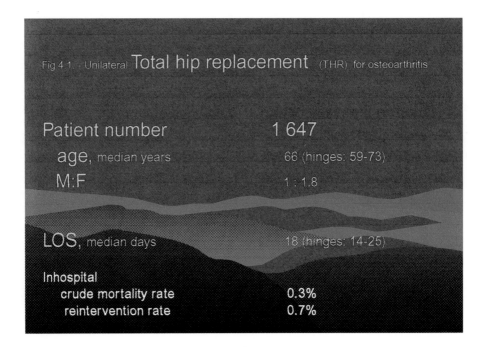

Fig 4.1. - Unilateral Total hip replacement (THR) for osteoarthritis

Patient number	1 647
age, median years	66 (hinges: 59-73)
M:F	1 : 1.8
LOS, median days	18 (hinges: 14-25)
Inhospital	
crude mortality rate	0.3%
reintervention rate	0.7%

I. Patient data and some variables related to surgery

Table 4.1 shows, by hospital, the number, age and gender of patients, and the values of some variables related to surgery. Age of patients was 65 to 70 years in two thirds of the hospitals (median values) and the modal M:F ratio was 1:2.5.

A preoperative Hct value was available in 90% of patients. The median value was 40% (hinges: 37-43%). The low values observed in two hospitals were associated with the donation of two to three PABD units by most of the patients operated there.

Table 4.1. THR: patient data and some variables related to surgery

	EA*	ID	EB*	GRD	GRF	PB	DKA	GRA	FC	EC	GBI	GBF	GBH	ED*	IB	IG	IH*	IL	FA	NLB	NLA	BA	GBC	DA*	IE*	DKB	DB	IC	DKC	BB	BC
Patient number	4	64	10	92	62	22	63	80	59	58	68	64	72	12	108	55	13	38	41	76	63	77	72	16	10	63	40	71	62	54	58
Age																															
median years	•	65	67	63	65	63	67	58	70	64	67	65	69	62	63	69	65	64	68	69	72	66	68	77	68	72	70	64	70	64	68
range	57-75	38-87	56-78	28-82	30-85	35-82	31-90	23-80	41-89	35-90	43-89	41-85	35-87	39-70	39-91	39-87	51-80	44-84	32-82	43-85	45-90	23-83	37-84	42-91	57-81	44-90	21-87	47-81	18-89	21-91	39-88
M:F ratio	1.0	0.4	1.0	0.2	0.4	1.4	0.6	0.4	0.8	0.7	1.3	0.5	0.4	0.7	0.3	0.5	1.6	1.4	0.8	0.5	0.4	0.5	0.6	0.2	0.7	0.9	0.6	0.5	0.3	0.8	0.4
Preoperative Hct																															
% Po with	75	97	100	87	97	100	95	93	100	33	71	67	90	33	84	100	85	95	100	100	98	100	93	94	90	97	92	84	98	100	100
median %	39	39	39	42	43	43	39	40	41	42	41	40	40	•	36	39	36	39	41	41	40	40	41	40	42	40	42	38	38	38	39
range	41-47	31-48	35-47	32-53	35-58	35-50	32-49	28-49	31-49	34-49	33-48	31-47	32-49	40-46	27-46	32-48	32-42	32-48	29-52	36-51	33-49	25-51	32-50	29-47	36-47	25-48	29-49	33-48	30-51	31-46	29-52
Drugs[1]																															
% Po	•	89	80	91		45	22	100	95	98	94	86	46	100	83	100	69	100	98	100	100	100	68	100	20	98	100	20	71	44	100
Anaesthesia, regional or combined																															
% Po		3		1	97		25	32		36	19	12	43			100		100		38	79	6	61		40	63	67		45	13	9
Duration of surgery																															
% Po with	100		100	18	42	100	67	60		100	62	56	67	100	57	14	100		100	74	48	79	81	100	100	54		100	69	74	69
median minutes			130	120	150	180	110	100		180	130	135	90	120	90	•	120			60	99	135	95		100	105		90	105	180	92
range			70-175	100-180	105-240	120-240	70-275	50-145		95-260	85-235	65-315	50-130	100-130	50-180		90-165			35-170	99-99	60-200	55-150		90-120	50-190		75-100	40-215	70-270	50-195
Blood loss																															
perioperative																															
% Po with	100	9	100				100	16	86	12	87	34	82	17	91	85			100	96	94	22	100	94	70	98	82	100	97	93	93
median L	•	•	0.4				0.6	0.6	0.6	0.7	0.8	0.6	0.6	•	0.6	0.7			1.0	0.4	0.6	0.6	0.4	0.5	0.3	0.7	1.5	0.4	1.1	0.8	0.4
range	0.2-1.8	0.2-1.3	0.2-1.1				0.1-4.8	0.5-2.1	0.2-2.2	0.3-1.0	0.1-2.0	0.2-2.0	0.2-1.6	0.4-0.5	0.1-3.0	0.3-2.0			0.4-2.4	0.1-1.6	0.1-1.8	0.1-2.1	0.1-1.8	0.3-1.5	0.3-0.8	0.1-2.2	0.2-7.0	0.0-1.3	0.1-5.9	0.2-2.0	0.1-1.1
postoperative																															
% Po with	25	58					3	15	91	83	96	95	18	16	33	76	61		100	88	76	100	95		93	60		93	97	92	90
median L	•	0.3					•	0.1	0.2	0.7	0.8	0.6	0.3	•	0.3	0.5	0.5		0.7	0.3	0.4	0.4	0.5		0.2		1.0	0.2	1.1	0.4	0.5
range	0.1-1.4						0.0-0.6	0.0-0.6	0.0-1.2	0.0-1.6	0.1-4.3	0.0-4.3	0.2-0.6	•	0.1-1.1	0.1-1.0	0.1-1.0		0.2-2.9	0.0-0.9	0.2-1.0	0.1-2.0	0.0-1.5		0.0-0.6		0.4-3.0	0.0-0.6		0.0-1.6	0.2-1.3

Po = patients operated.
[1] Only anticoagulants were administered.
• = not calculated due to the small sample size.
Hospital code and * = less than 20 patients.

78% of patients received a drug acting on the coagulation system: 34% both before and after surgery, 27% only after surgery and 17% only before. Drugs (Figure 4.2) administered before surgery were mainly low-dose heparin (13%), aspirin and NSAID (8%), and those given after surgery were low-dose heparin (50%), coumarin (6%) and heparin anticoagulant dose (0.8%); in 4% of patients the type of drug was not specified.

Anaesthesia was general in 69%, regional in 25% and combined in 6% of patients. In two hospitals (IG, IL) only regional anaesthesia was used and in four other hospitals (GRF, NLA, GBC, DB) regional or combined anaesthesia was normally used.

Information on duration of surgery was available in 54% of patients. The median time was 110 minutes (hinges: 90-140) and varied among hospitals by a factor of three. It is not known whether these differences were genuine or attributable to different ways of recording duration of procedure.

Perioperative and postoperative blood loss were documented in 64 and 54% of patients, respectively. The median volumes were 0.6 L (hinges: 0.4-1.0) and 0.47 L (hinges: 0.3-0.7), respectively. According to recorded perioperative blood loss, 7% of patients bled more than 1.5 L (Figure 4.3).

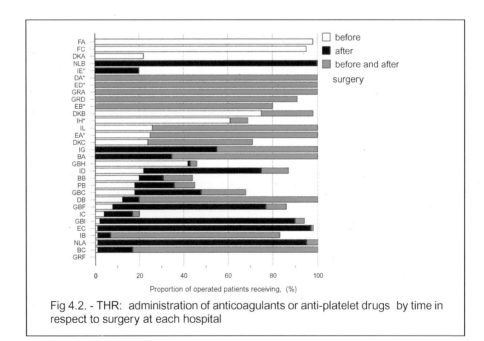

Fig 4.2. - THR: administration of anticoagulants or anti-platelet drugs by time in respect to surgery at each hospital

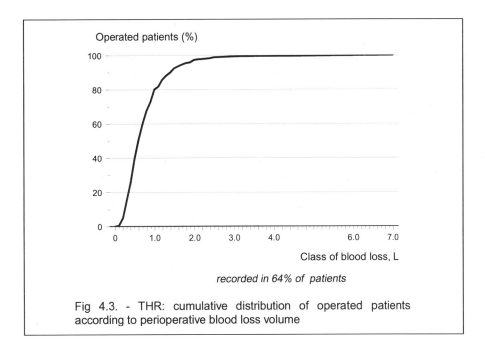

Fig 4.3. - THR: cumulative distribution of operated patients according to perioperative blood loss volume

II. Transfusion data

Detailed transfusion data are given by hospital in Table 4.2. The majority (16) of the hospitals used blood components together with albumin and artificial colloids, 11 of these were in the central-northern European area. Hospitals in Belgium, Germany, and the Netherlands used a similar combination of products.

II.1.0. *Red units*

In all 1 331 patients (81%) were transfused with 4 526 red units. The proportion of patients transfused varied from 29 to 100% among hospitals. In hospitals of central-northern Europe, it was less than half that in hospitals of the Mediterranean area (RR = 0.4 (0.3 to 0.6)).

In transfused patients, the median number of units given was three (hinges: 2-4). In about half of the hospitals, the median was two and in the remainder from 2.5 to five. Of operated patients, 16% received more than four red units (Figure 4.4).

II.1.1. *Allogeneic and autologous transfusion of red units*

In all 935 patients were transfused with 3 048 allogeneic units, 257 with 779 autologous units and 139 with 384 autologous and 315 allogeneic units (Figure 4.5). The use of allogeneic and autologous units by hospital is shown in Figure 4.6. In hospitals of central-northern Europe, the percentage of patients transfused with autologous red units was much lower than in hospitals of the Mediterranean area (RR = 0.03 (0.01 to 0.12)).

Table 4.2. THR: transfusion data

	EA*	ID	EB*	GRD	GRF	PB	DKA	GRA	FC	EC	GBI	GBF	GBH	ED*	IB	IG	IH*	IL	FA	NLB	NLA	BA	GBC	DA*	IE*	DKB	DB	IC	DKC	BB	BC
Red units																															
patients																															
transfused/operated (%)	50	65.6	70	100	100	100	80.9	87.5	35.6	81	82.3	87.5	88.9	91.7	100	100	100	100	29.3	46	52.4	58.4	70.8	75	80	82.5	87.5	90.1	93.5	96.3	98.3
units per transfused patient																															
median	•	2		4	4	2	3	3	2	2	3	3	2	•	5	3	•	2	2	2	2	2	2	•	•	2.5	4	3	4	4	4
hinges	2-3	2-3		4-5	4-5	2-3	2-5	2-4	2-3	2-3	2-4	2-3	2-3	•	3-7	2-4	•	2-3	1-2.5	2-2	1-2	2-3	2-3	•	•	2-4	2-5	2-4	3-5	2-4.5	3-5
Plasma																															
patients																															
transfused/operated (%)	1.5			16.3	30.6	95.4		2.5	1.7	1.7					1			63.2			1.6			6.2			7.5		6.4	9.3	12.1
units per transfused patient																															
median	•			2	2	2		•	•	•					•			2			•			•			•		•	•	2
hinges				1-2	1-2	1-2												2-2													2-2
Platelets																															
patients																															
transfused/operated (%)				1.1												1.8													1.6		
Albumin																															
patients																															
administered/operated (%)							76.2	1.2											4.9	1.3	23.8	61	2.8	6.2	10	28.6	20	2.8	22.6	40.7	56.9
grams per recipient																															
median							26												•		21	41		•	•	21	9.5	•	13	21	21
hinges							13-38														21-26	41-61				13-26	6-17.5		13-26	21-41	21-41
Colloids																															
patients																															
administered/operated (%)									96.6	3.4	25	28.1	75	16.7	2.8	76.4	23.1	89.5	97.6	84.2	98.4	48	48.6	62.5	30	88.9	82.5	95.8	95.2	94.4	96.5
L per recipient																															
median									1.5	•	0.5	0.5	0.5	•	•	1.25	•	1	1.5	0.5	0.5	1	0.5	•		0.5	0.5	1	0.5	2.5	1.5
hinges									1-1.5		0.5-1	0.5-0.5	0.5-1			0.5-2		0.5-1	1-2.0	0.5-1	0.5-0.5	1-1.5	0.5-1			0.5-0.5	0.3-1	0.5-1	0.5-1	1-2.5	0.5-2.5
Patients for whom the number of autologous blood units was not reported (% Po)																							1.4								

Hospitals are aggregated according to products used.

◇ identifies hospitals where autotransfusion was used.

* identifies hospitals where less than 20 patients are available.

• identifies hospitals where the values were not calculated due to the small sample size.

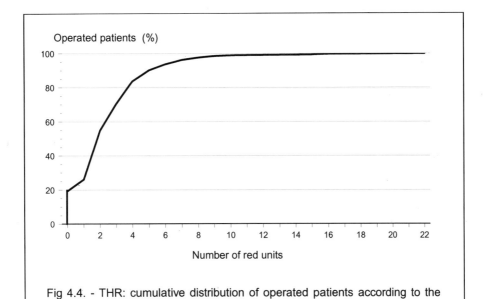

Fig 4.4. - THR: cumulative distribution of operated patients according to the number of red units transfused

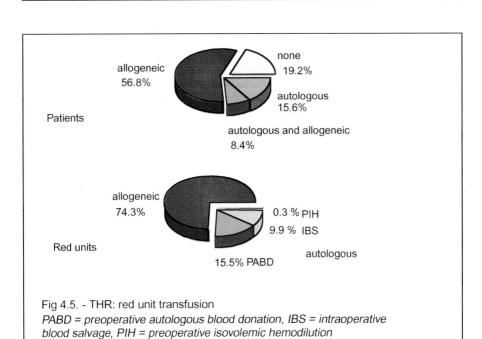

Fig 4.5. - THR: red unit transfusion
PABD = preoperative autologous blood donation, IBS = intraoperative blood salvage, PIH = preoperative isovolemic hemodilution

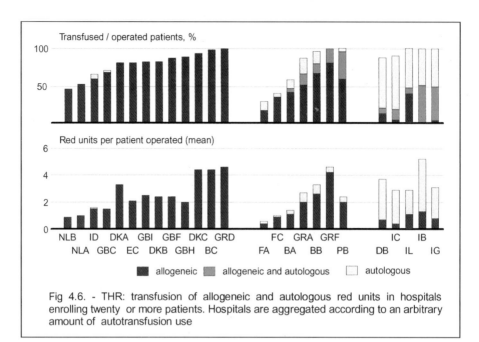

Fig 4.6. - THR: transfusion of allogeneic and autologous red units in hospitals enrolling twenty or more patients. Hospitals are aggregated according to an arbitrary amount of autotransfusion use

PABD was the most widely used autotransfusion technique (Figure 4.7). It provided 1.5 times more units than were provided by all the other techniques (Figure 4.5). Autotransfusion techniques were used in about half of the hospitals. Figure 4.7 also shows that a greater use of autotransfusion techniques was associated with an increased proportion of patients receiving autologous blood.

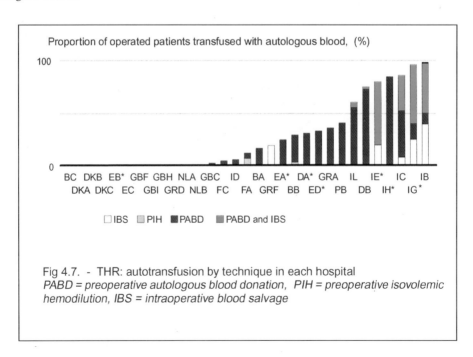

Fig 4.7. - THR: autotransfusion by technique in each hospital
PABD = preoperative autologous blood donation, PIH = preoperative isovolemic hemodilution, IBS = intraoperative blood salvage

In hospitals with no or low autotransfusion use, a correlation was found between the proportion of transfused patients and the number of red units per recipient (Figure 4.8), suggesting that when more patients are transfused more units are also given.

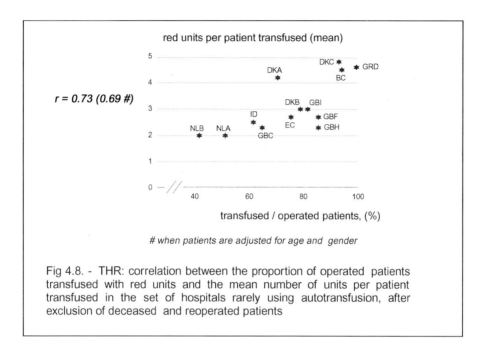

Fig 4.8. - THR: correlation between the proportion of operated patients transfused with red units and the mean number of units per patient transfused in the set of hospitals rarely using autotransfusion, after exclusion of deceased and reoperated patients

Data on the proportion of transfused patients and the mean number of units given per patient transfused, comparing the Sanguis study findings and published reports, is shown in Figure 4.9. The majority of the Sanguis hospitals had a blood use within the range of the published reports, while in about one third, blood use was greater.

II.1.2. *Allogeneic whole blood use*

Of transfused red units, 31% were given as whole blood. Half or more of the red units transfused in three Greek hospitals, two British and one Spanish hospital (Figure 4.10) were whole blood.

II.1.3. *Time of transfusion*

Transfusion episodes occurred predominantly during the day of surgery and progressively decreased in frequency during the first five days after operation (Figure 4.11). Postoperative transfusion (Figure 4.12) affected one third to a half of patients in some hospitals (Belgian hospitals, FC, DKA, IB).

The mean number of transfusion episodes per patient transfused was 1.7.

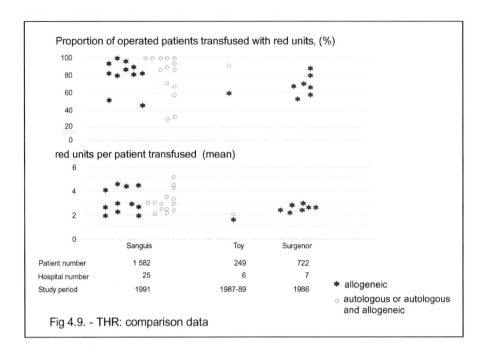

Fig 4.9. - THR: comparison data

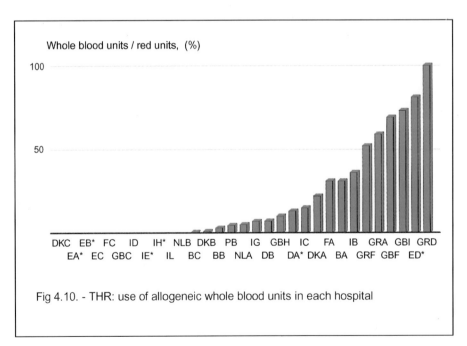

Fig 4.10. - THR: use of allogeneic whole blood units in each hospital

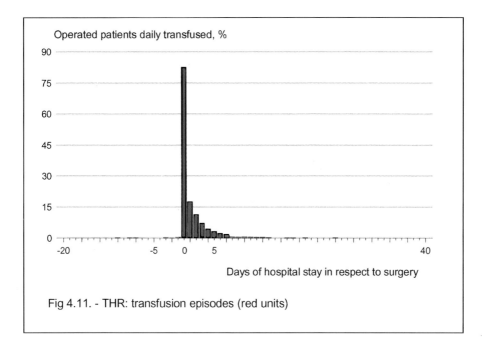

Fig 4.11. - THR: transfusion episodes (red units)

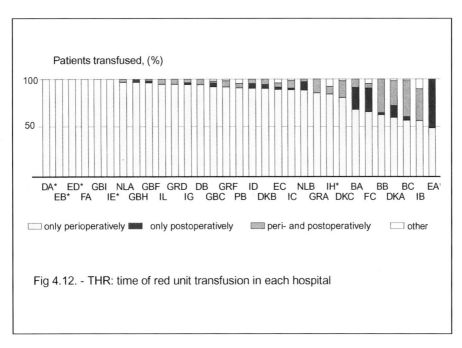

Fig 4.12. - THR: time of red unit transfusion in each hospital

II.2.0. *Plasma*

In all 215 plasma units were transfused to 106 (6%) patients in more than half of the hospitals (Figure 4.13). The percentage of plasma recipients in the hospitals of central-northern Europe, although lower, did not significantly differ from that in the hospitals of the Mediterranean area (RR = 0.8 (0.1 to 4.0)).

In transfused patients the median number of plasma units was two (hinges: 1-2).

Fifty plasma units (23%) were autologous and were transfused to 25 patients in three hospitals (BB, DB, IL, the latter hospital accounting for 42 units). Of the remaining units, 111 (52%) were fresh frozen, seven (3%) from apheresis (BC) and 47 (22%) liquid (hospitals EC, IB, NLA, PB, the latter accounting for 42 liquid units).

Fifty-one patients received allogeneic plasma along with red units, 48 of them within the same 24-hour period.

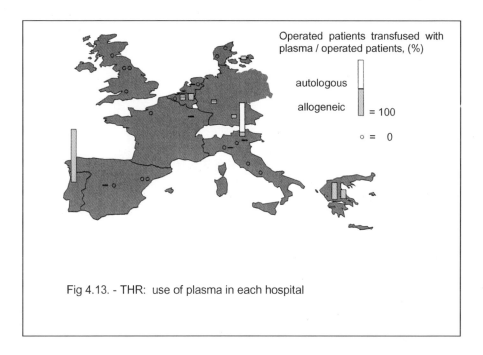

Fig 4.13. - THR: use of plasma in each hospital

II.3.0. *Albumin*

In all 215 patients (13%) received 7 147 g of albumin. Albumin was transfused in about half of the hospitals, two thirds of them in central-northern Europe (Figure 4.14). In these hospitals, the percentage of albumin recipients was three times that in hospitals of the Mediterranean area (RR = 3 (1 to 10)). In recipients, the median quantity given was 26 g (hinges: 21-41). Hospitals using albumin differed widely in both the percentage of recipients (1 to 76%) and in the amount used (range of the medians 9 to 41 g). A high use of albumin was seen in a few hospitals (BA, BC, DKA), in which 59% of the recipients and 68% of the total amount given were observed.

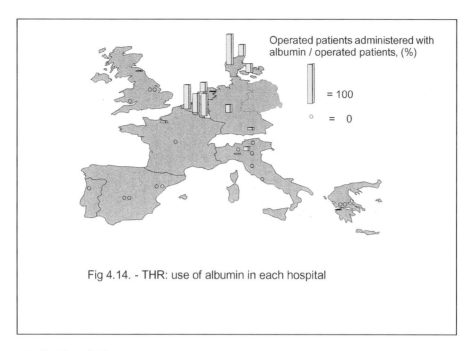

Fig 4.14. - THR: use of albumin in each hospital

II.4.0. *Artificial colloids*

In all 914 L of artificial colloids were administered to 806 patients (49%) in three quarters of the hospitals (Figure 4.15). The median volume was 0.5 L (hinges: 0.5-1.2). A high use of artificial colloids was observed in some hospitals, the majority of them was in central-northern Europe. Consequently, the proportion of recipients in hospitals of central-northern Europe was much higher than that in the Mediterranean area (RR = 68 (27 to 174)).

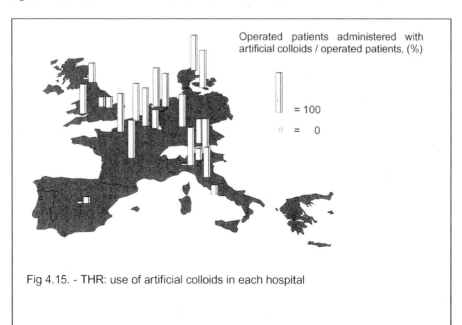

Fig 4.15. - THR: use of artificial colloids in each hospital

The variability among hospitals in the type of colloid used and the amount per operated patients is shown in Figure 4.16. In recipients, the median volume of dextran and HES varied among hospitals from 0.5 to 1.2 L, and that of gelatin from 0.6 to 1.8 L.

The variation in the clinical use of products in the hospitals studied is shown in Figure 4.17 and that in hospitals aggregated according to country in Figure 4.18.

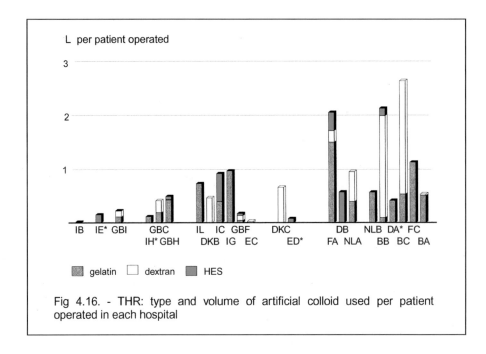

Fig 4.16. - THR: type and volume of artificial colloid used per patient operated in each hospital

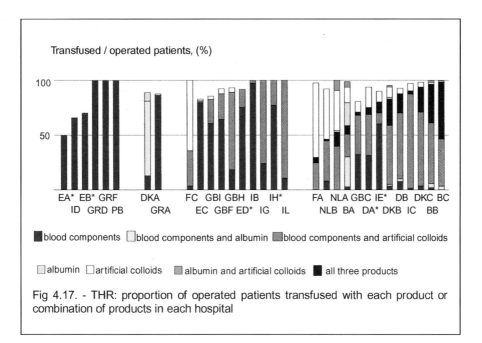

Fig 4.17. - THR: proportion of operated patients transfused with each product or combination of products in each hospital

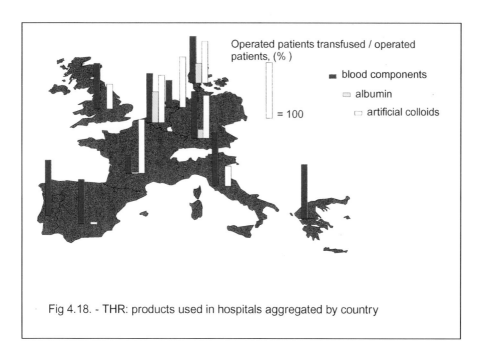

Fig 4.18. - THR: products used in hospitals aggregated by country

III. Reasons for transfusion documented in the medical record

III.1. *Red units*

A reason was documented in 23% of the recipients (Figure 4.19) and in 22 of 31 hospitals. Documentation was more frequent in hospitals of the central-northern European area.

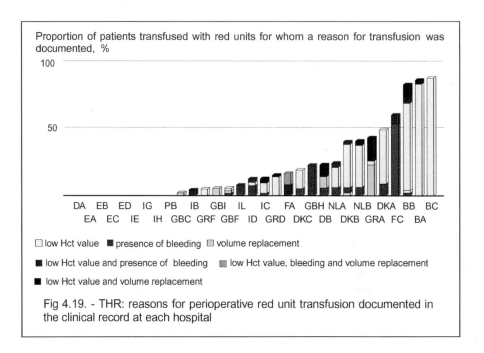

Fig 4.19. - THR: reasons for perioperative red unit transfusion documented in the clinical record at each hospital

III.2. *Plasma*

Reasons were given for 7% of recipients from four hospitals. In 4% of recipients they were volume replacement, bleeding or both.

III.3. *Albumin*

Reasons were given for 1% of recipients from two hospitals.

III.4. *Artificial colloids*

Reasons (volume replacement) were given for 7% of patients from five hospitals.

IV. Variables associated with red unit transfusion

IV.1. *Transfused versus untransfused patients*

The profiles of untransfused and transfused patients are shown in Table 4.3. Untransfused patients were in a higher proportion males, had a slightly higher preoperative Hct value and a

114

lower blood loss than patients transfused with allogeneic units, even after exclusion of re-operated and deceased patients. Approximately 70% of untransfused patients were from certain hospitals (NLA, NLB, FA, FC, BA, GBC, ID). Patients transfused with autologous red units were younger than transfused patients, and had a lower preoperative Hct value attributable to predonation. Of patients transfused with autologous red units, 75% were from certain hospitals (IB, IC, IL, IG, GRA, GRF, DB). A high reoperation rate and a high number of units transfused characterized the sub-set of patients who were transfused with autologous and allogeneic red units.

Table 4.3. THR: comparison between patients transfused and not transfused with red units during the hospital stay

	Patients transfused			Patients not transfused	95% confidence interval of the difference[2]
	allogeneic	allogeneic and autologous	autologous		
Patient number	935	139	257	316	
Age, years[1]	68 (60-75)	64 (57-71)	63 (56-70)	67 (59-72)	−0.4 to 2.4
M:F	*0.44*	0.39	0.6	*0.9*	*13 to 25*
Hct preintervention, %[1]	*40 (37-43)*	38 (35-41)	38 (35-41)	*42 (40-45)*	*1.7 to 2.7*
Percentage of patients with	88	91	91	94	
Anaesthesia, regional and/or combined, % Po	31	34	31	31	
Anticoagulants, % Po	77	73	73	89	
Duration of surgery, min[1]	120 (95-150)	120 (90-150)	95 (90-120)	99 (80-120)	
Percentage of patients with	56	60	51	50	
Blood loss, L[1]	*0.7 (0.5-1.0)*	0.7 (0.5-1.2)	0.6 (0.4-0.9)	*0.5 (0.3-0.7)*	*0.6 to 0.7*[3]
Percentage of patients with	36	65	69	71	
Red units per patient transfused[1]	3 (2-5)	4 (3-6)	2 (2-3)		
Stated reason for transfusion, % Pt	28	22	11		
Percentage of patients transfused with					
plasma	6.4	16.5	8.2		
albumin	16.5	5.7	6.6	11.4	
artificial colloids	46.5	32.4	54.9	58.5	
		100	100		
Reintervention for bleeding, % Po	0.53	3.6	0.39		
In-hospital crude mortality rate, % Po	0.43			0.31	
Last Hct, %[1]	33 (31-36)	31 (29-33)	31 (29-34)	33 (30-35)	
Percentage of patients with	87	93	94	92	
Hospital stay, number of days[1]	17 (14-24)	26 (20-34)	23 (18-28)	15 (12-19)	
before surgery	2 (1-5)	6 (3-12)	6 (3-11)	2 (1-3)	
after surgery	14 (12-18)	18 (14-22)	15 (13-19)	13 (11-16)	

Po = patients operated.
Pt = patients transfused.
[1] Median (hinges).
[2] Between patients not transfused and transfused with allogeneic units, after exclusion of deaths and reinterventions.
[3] Performed on ln values.
Note: *significant differences are shown in bold italics.*

IV.2. *Preoperative transfusion*

Twenty-two patients (1%) were transfused with a mean of 2.5 red units before surgery. A striking event, occurring in 14 patients, was the re-transfusion before surgery of predonated autologous blood units that were set aside for the operation. A hospital effect was observed: 11 of these patients were from one hospital (IB). A pretransfusion Hct value was recorded in only eight of these and the median value was 30% (range 28 to 41%). Before surgery, the post-transfusion Hct was available in half of the patients and the median value was 34% (range 28 to 39%).

IV.3. *Perioperative patient transfusion*

Indicator: proportion of operated patients perioperatively transfused with red units (mean percentage ± SE)
Hospitals: 16 (64%) of 25 enrolling 20 or more patients
Patients: 1 019 (62%) of 1 631, after exclusion of deaths and reinterventions
Variables: age, gender, preoperative Hct, blood loss, type of anaesthesia, use of anticoagulants, use of autotransfusion

Since the effect of a variable on the probability of a patient being transfused cannot be estimated when all or nearly all patients (90% or more) are transfused, one third of the hospitals with this feature were not analysed. No systematic differences were found in age, gender, preoperative Hct and blood loss distributions in patients of hospitals included and not included in the analysis. The use of autotransfusion was higher in hospitals excluded from analysis.

On average, the probability of a patient being transfused was not affected by age (Part I, Figure 0.14), administration of anticoagulants (65% ± 1.4 both without and with anticoagulants), or anaesthesia (regional 61% ± 2.1, combined 62% ± 3.3, general 71% ± 1.1). It was higher in females (+ 17%) than in males. Furthermore, the higher the preoperative Hct, the lower the probability of transfusion (difference between the highest and lowest class of Hct = − 23%), whereas the higher the blood loss, the higher the probability of transfusion (difference between the highest and lowest class of blood loss = + 32%).

The probability of a patient being transfused was higher in hospitals with a high use of autotransfusion compared with those that rarely use autotransfusion (88% ± 1.6 versus 67% ± 0.7). Furthermore, in hospitals with a high use of autotransfusion, transfusion was rather independent of the effect of preoperative Hct and blood loss. In these hospitals, the probability of a patient being transfused, even with preoperative Hct values of 42% or higher, or with blood loss of 0.5 L or lower, was nearly twice that in the hospitals not using autotransfusion. Both observations suggest that criteria for transfusion of autologous blood may be substantially different from those used for allogeneic blood.

Age affected patient transfusion in nine of 16 hospitals (but in two cases younger patients were transfused more than the older), gender in nine of 16 hospitals, preoperative Hct in 11 of 16 hospitals (Figure 4.20) (in one case the trend was contradictory), and blood loss in 10 of 11 hospitals (Figure 4.21) (in one case contradictory).

116

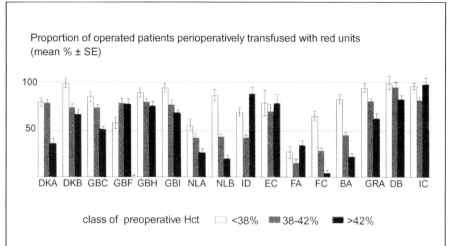

Fig 4.20. - THR: effect of preoperative Hct on the proportion of patients perioperatively transfused with red units in each hospital, after adjustment for age and gender

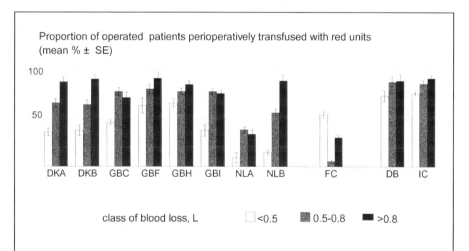

Fig 4.21. - THR: effect of blood loss on the proportion of patients perioperatively transfused with red units in each hospital, after adjustment for age and gender

117

Hospitals were observed where most of the studied factors affected patient transfusion in a comprehensible way, whereas in others a rationale based on the examined variables could be discerned in part (Figure 4.22).

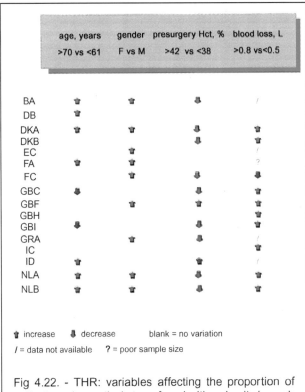

	age, years >70 vs <61	gender F vs M	presurgery Hct, % >42 vs <38	blood loss, L >0.8 vs<0.5
BA	⬆	⬆	⬇	/
DB	⬆			
DKA	⬆	⬆	⬇	⬆
DKB			⬇	⬆
EC		⬆		/
FA	⬆	⬆		?
FC		⬆	⬇	⬇
GBC	⬇		⬇	⬆
GBF		⬆	⬆	⬆
GBH				⬆
GBI	⬇		⬇	⬆
GRA		⬆	⬇	/
IC				⬆
ID	⬆		⬆	/
NLA	⬆	⬆	⬇	⬆
NLB	⬆	⬆	⬇	⬆

⬆ increase   ⬇ decrease   blank = no variation
/ = data not available   ? = poor sample size

Fig 4.22. - THR: variables affecting the proportion of patients perioperatively transfused with red units in each hospital. The comparison is performed between the highest and lowest class of each variable in each hospital

The probability of a patient being transfused still differed among hospitals after adjustment for age, gender and preoperative Hct (Figure 4.23): from 24% ±2.1 to 93% ±1.4 (difference = 69%). Further adjustment for blood loss still left remarkable interhospital differences (Figure 4.24), i.e. from 37% ±5.7 to 87% ±4.6 (difference = 50%).

In ascending order, differences in the proportion of patients transfused attributable to gender were 17%, to preoperative Hct value 23%, to blood loss 32%, and to other unknown factors associated with the individual hospital 50%.

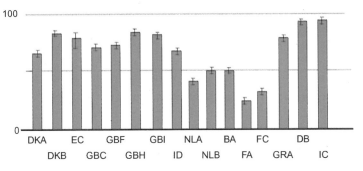

Proportion of operated patients perioperatively transfused with red units
(mean % ± SE)

Fig 4.23. - THR: probability of a patient being perioperatively transfused with red units in each hospital, after adjustment for age, gender and preoperative Hct

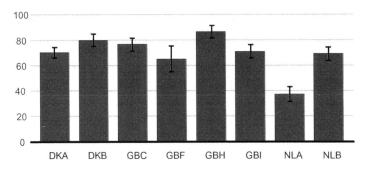

Proportion of operated patients perioperatively transfused with red units
(mean % ± SE)

Fig 4.24. - THR: probability of a patient being perioperatively transfused with red units in each hospital, after adjustment for age, gender, preoperative Hct and blood loss

119

The relative role of blood loss and preoperative Hct in initiating the decision to transfuse perioperatively can be seen also in Figure 4.25. When blood loss was higher than 0.8 L, about 80% of Patients were transfused regardless of their preoperative Hct value; when between 0.5 and 0.8 L, about 60% were transfused when preoperative Hct was higher than 42%. When blood loss was less than 0.5 L, the proportion of patients transfused was as low as about 40% but only in patients whose preoperative Hct was equal to or higher than 38%.

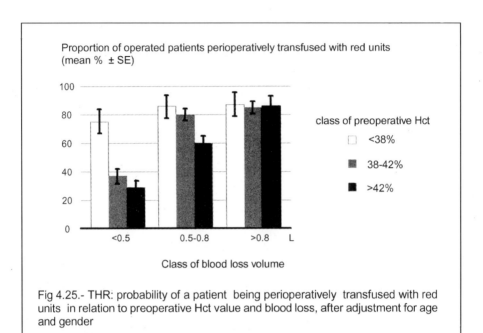

Fig 4.25.- THR: probability of a patient being perioperatively transfused with red units in relation to preoperative Hct value and blood loss, after adjustment for age and gender

The association between duration of surgery and blood loss was studied in 593 patients from 21 hospitals. Table 4.4 reports the results obtained.

Table 4.4. Distribution of duration of surgery by blood loss category

Blood loss, L	Duration of surgery, minutes		
	< 100	100-120	> 120
	percentage of patients		
> 0.8	26	32	42
0.5-0.8	46	29	25
< 0.5	66	20	14

Of patients with a blood loss lower than 0.5 L, 66% had a duration of surgery lower than 100 minutes, whereas 42% of patients with a blood loss higher than 0.8 L had a duration of surgery higher than 120 minutes. A positive association appeared between duration of surgery and perioperative blood loss. No firm conclusion can be drawn because it cannot be excluded that the ways in which duration of surgery was recorded might differ among hospitals.

The relationship between perioperative blood loss volumes and anticoagulants (administered up to surgery) was also considered in 783 patients (Table 4.5). There seemed to be no association.

Table 4.5. Distribution of blood loss by use of anticoagulants

	Blood loss, L		
	<0.5	0.5-0.8	>0.8
Anticoagulant	percentage of patients		
yes	26	39	35
no	40	35	25

IV.4. *Perioperative red unit transfusion*

Indicator: red units per patient perioperatively transfused (mean number ± SE per patient transfused)
Hospitals: 25 (100%) of 25 enrolling 20 or more patients
Patients: 1 218 (75%) of 1 631, after exclusion of deaths and reinterventions
Factors: age, gender, preintervention Hct, blood loss, use of autologous units, use of anticoagulants, type of anaesthesia

On average (Table 4.6), the mean number of units transfused was not affected by age, gender, type of anaesthesia (regional 2.3 ± 0.06, combined 2.5 ± 0.09, general 2.4 ± 0.04), whereas it was slightly higher in females than in males, and with the use of anticoagulants (2.5 ± 0.06 versus 3.0 ± 0.03). Furthermore, the higher the blood loss, the higher the number of units transfused (difference between the highest and lowest class of blood loss = + 1.4), the higher the preoperative Hct, the slightly lower the number of units transfused (difference between the highest and lowest class of preoperative Hct = − 0.6).

The mean number of units per patient transfused was slightly higher in hospitals with a high use of autotransfusion when compared to those with no use (3.3 ± 0.10 versus 2.8 ± 0.05); furthermore the number of units decreased with increasing preoperative Hct (from 4.4 ± 0.17 to 2.5 ± 0.16 versus 2.9 ± 0.09 to 2.7 ± 0.06), and with decreasing blood loss (from 5.2 ± 0.09 to 2.9 ± 0.12 versus 2.9 ± 0.07 to 2.2 ± 0.10) only in hospitals with high autotransfusion use.

In ascending order, differences in the number of units transfused attributable to preoperative Hct value were 0.6 units, to blood loss 1.4 units, while to other, unknown factors associated to the hospital 3.5 units.

After adjustment for age, gender, preoperative Hct and blood loss, the number of units transfused varied among hospitals from 1.4 ± 0.2 to 4.5 ± 0.2 (difference = 3.1) (Figure 4.26). Diversities were larger in hospitals with no use of autotransfusion than in those with high autotransfusion use (1.6 ± 0.4 to 4.4 ± 0.2 versus 3.4 ± 0.2 to 4.5 ± 0.2).

Table 4.6. THR: effect of some variables on the number of red units per patient transfused in each hospital (mean ± SE)

Hospital	Patient number	Factor first, third tertile (or category): Global [1]	Age, years [2] <61	Age, years [2] >70	Gender [2] F	Gender [2] M	Preintervention Hct, % [1] <38	Preintervention Hct, % [1] >42	Blood loss, L [1] <0.5	Blood loss, L [1] >0.8
Autotransfusion <10%										
BC	53	3.7±0.11	2.8±0.19	3.6±0.20					2.9±0.19	5.8±0.42
DKA	44	3.2±0.07	2.2±0.12	4.8±0.10	3.7±0.07	2.8±0.12	4.9±0.12	4.0±0.22	1.3±0.19	4.7±0.14
DKB	50	3.1±0.07	3.4±0.18	2.5±0.08	3.3±0.10	2.9±0.09			2.3±0.22	3.4±0.11
DKC	58	4.1±0.10	3.7±0.18	5.1±0.17			4.6±0.20	2.9±0.24	1.2±0.63	5.0±0.17
GBC	47	2.1±0.06			2.4±0.08	1.8±0.10			2.1±0.12	2.8±0.20
GBF	55	2.8±0.06	2.9±0.08	2.5±0.10						
GBH	61	2.2±0.06			2.2±0.07	2.3±0.10	2.6±0.17	3.2±0.14		
GBI	55	3.0±0.06			2.6±0.08	3.4±0.07	2.2±0.12	1.7±0.11	2.0±0.17	2.7±0.13
GRD	92	4.5±0.09								
NLA	32	1.4±0.18								
NLB	32	1.9±0.10								
ID	39	2.4±0.08	2.6±0.11	2.0±0.13						
EC	44	2.5±0.07	2.9±0.11	2.4±0.14						
	662	2.8±0.05	2.7±0.02	3.0±0.02	3.0±0.01	2.7±0.02	2.9±0.09	2.7±0.06	2.2±0.10	2.9±0.07
Autotransfusion between 10 and 50%										
BB	51	2.8±0.04	2.5±0.06	3.1±0.07	3.2±0.05	2.5±0.06	2.8±0.05	3.8±0.17	2.9±0.11	5.5±0.08
BA	35	2.4±0.06								
FA	12	1.8±0.19					2.3±0.26	0.8±0.26		
FC	15	3.0±0.11	5.2±0.28	2.4±0.16	3.6±0.16	2.4±0.23	2.2±0.19	6.3±0.41		
GRF	62	4.5±0.03	5.0±0.06	4.2±0.07			6.1±0.17	4.5±0.05		
GRA	70	2.6±0.04					3.2±0.12	1.7±0.13		
PB	21	2.5±0.06			2.9±0.05	2.3±0.07				
	266	2.8±0.08	3.2±0.03	2.8±0.04	3.0±0.02	2.6±0.04	3.1±0.09	3.1±0.09	1.9±0.31	2.9±0.45
Autotransfusion > 50%										
DB	34	3.9±0.16					6.2±0.46	2.5±0.25	3.3±0.35	4.4±0.12
IB	107	4.2±0.04			4.4±0.04	4.1±0.07	4.5±0.17	3.2±0.36	3.1±0.13	6.6±0.10
IG	54	3.1±0.05	3.5±0.10	2.8±0.09			4.5±0.28	2.8±0.28	2.7±0.18	4.5±0.11
IL	37	2.8±0.06	2.0±0.12	4.0±0.11	2.5±0.10	3.1±0.08	3.6±0.38	1.6±0.48		
IC	58	2.8±0.12					3.1±0.19	2.0±0.34	2.3±0.09	4.9±0.25
	290	3.3±0.1	3.4±0.04	3.5±0.04	3.4±0.03	3.3±0.01	4.4±0.17	2.5±0.16	2.9±0.12	5.2±0.09
Total	1 218	2.9±0.01	3.0±0.02	3.0±0.02	3.1±0.01	2.8±0.01	3.3±0.05	2.7±0.04	2.3±0.08	3.7±0.06

Blank = no variation.
[1] After adjustment for both age and gender.
[2] Age was adjusted for gender, and gender for age.

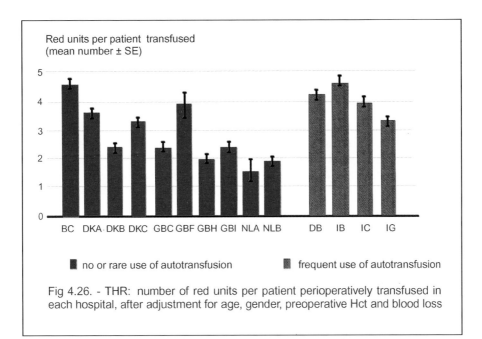

Fig 4.26. - THR: number of red units per patient perioperatively transfused in each hospital, after adjustment for age, gender, preoperative Hct and blood loss

IV.5. *Postoperative transfusion*

After exclusion of deaths and reinterventions, 191 (11%) patients were postoperatively transfused. The average threshold for transfusion was an Hct value of 26% ± 3.1 (Table 4.7), to reach a post-transfusion value similar to that of untransfused patients. Records of post-transfusion Hct were found, however, in less than one third of patients. Nearly two thirds of patients transfused postoperatively were from certain hospitals (IB, BB, BC, DKA, DKC, GRA).

Table 4.7. THR: some characteristics of patients transfused and not transfused with red units in the postoperative period,[1] after exclusion of deaths and reinterventions

	Patients transfused	Patients not transfused	95% confidence interval of the difference
Patient number	191	1 440	
Age, years[2]	67 ± 12	65 ± 11	−4 to −0.3
Percentage of males	30	36	−0.8 to 13
Hct pretransfusion, %[2]	26 ± 3.1		
Percentage of patients with	48		
Postoperative blood loss, mL[3]	6.0 ± 1.1	6.0 ± 1.2	0.8 to 1.2
Percentage of patients with	74	54	
Units per patient transfused[2]	1.8 ± 0.8		
Last Hct, %[2]	33 ± 4.3	33 ± 4.3	−1.2 to 1.2
Percentage of patients with	28	88	
Postsurgical LOS, days[2]	19.7 ± 10	15.5 ± 6	

[1] From the fourth day after surgery to discharge.
[2] Means ± SD.
[3] Expressed as ln mean ± SD.

V. Some outcome data

Table 4.8 shows some outcome variables. In operated patients the last Hct value was available at a median number of six days (hinges: 2-10) after surgery; the median value was 33% (hinges: 30-35%). In nearly half of the hospitals the last Hct ranged from 28 to 31%, in one quarter 32 to 34%, and in the remaining quarter 35 to 36%.

In patients transfused with red units the last Hct was recorded after all transfusions were given five days (hinges: 2-10) after surgery; the median value was 33% (hinges: 30-36%). In a few hospitals (FA, IB, IC), 75% of patients had an Hct value lower than 33%, whereas in other hospitals (BC, GBH, GBI, NLB, GRF) 75% of patients had an Hct value higher than 33% (Figure 4.27). A small proportion of patients (0.6%) showed a value of the last Hct lower than 24%.

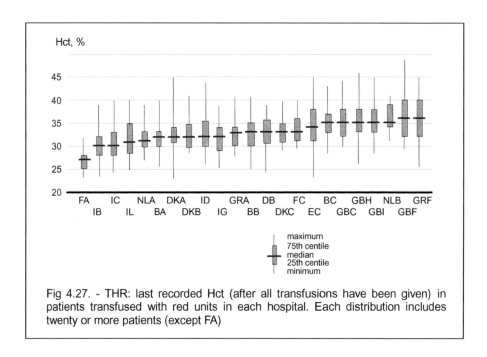

Fig 4.27. - THR: last recorded Hct (after all transfusions have been given) in patients transfused with red units in each hospital. Each distribution includes twenty or more patients (except FA)

Figures 4.28 and 4.29 show, by hospital, the mean Hct fall in both transfused and untransfused patients.

Recorded blood loss was compared with computed blood loss according to Toy *et al.* [5] Results obtained in each hospital for transfused and untransfused patients are illustrated in Figures 4.30 and 4.31, respectively.

The recorded blood loss was widely higher than that estimated. Only in four hospitals was the computed blood loss underestimated. In hospitals where the recorded blood loss did not exceed the computed loss by more than 0.4 L, recorded blood loss paralleled transfusion volumes when Hct fall was similar (Figure 4.32).

Table 4.8. THR: outcome variables

	EA*	ID	EB*	GRD	GRF	PB	DKA	GRA	FC	EC	GBI	GBF	GBH	ED*	IB	IG	IH*	IL	FA	NLB	NLA	BA	GBC	DA*	IE*	DKB	DB	IC	DKC	BB	BC
Last Hct																															
% Po with	89		100	55	77	36	100	90	98	83	73	81	93	100	98	96	61	95	100	99	87	97	85	81	100	92	97	97	100	100	100
(%) median	32		31	32	36	31	32	32	33	34	35	35	36	32	30	32	30	31	28	35	32	32	35	31	29	31	33	30	33	33	34
range	25-44		27-37	21-45	25-45	26-36	22-45	25-41	26-40	23-45	20-45	26-49	26-46	29-39	23-39	24-38	25-37	24-40	23-37	30-44	25-39	25-40	27-44	24-37	25-34	24-41	23-39	23-40	26-42	25-41	28-43
Complications of																															
allogeneic autologous transfusion (% Pt)					1.6		2.0	13.2				1.8								2.9		5.6								7.0 / 12.5	5.2
Reoperation																															
% Po	1.5						1.6			1.5								2.6			1.6						2.5	7.0			
Mortality																															
% Po													1.4														2.5			1.8	
LOS																															
median days	30		22	24	29	34	13	15	17	14	17	16	15	15	25	25	23	23	16	13	16	19	14	10	18	10	22	27	12	30	17
range	13-59		14-34	8-54	15-68	15-60	6-91	6-42	8-59	10-45	3-39	8-51	6-23	9-46	4-64	11-52	18-33	17-57	6-46	8-35	8-107	12-30	7-43	7-17	11-24	4-23	2-56	9-49	7-26	15-79	8-52

Po = patients operated.
Pt = patients transfused.
Hospital code and * = less than 20 patients.

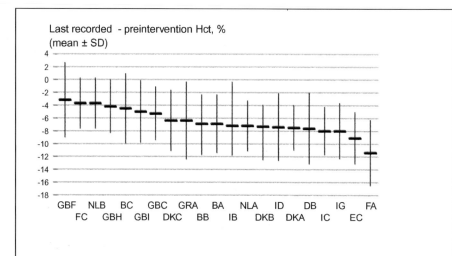

Fig 4.28. - THR: fall of Hct value in patients transfused with red units in each hospital

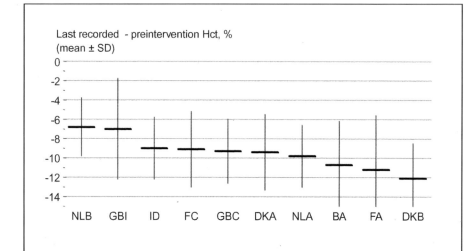

Fig 4.29. - THR: fall of Hct value in patients not transfused with red units in each hospital

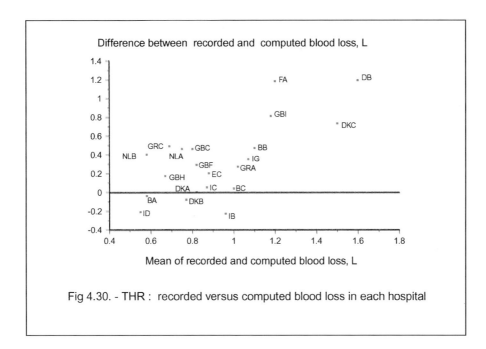

Fig 4.30. - THR : recorded versus computed blood loss in each hospital

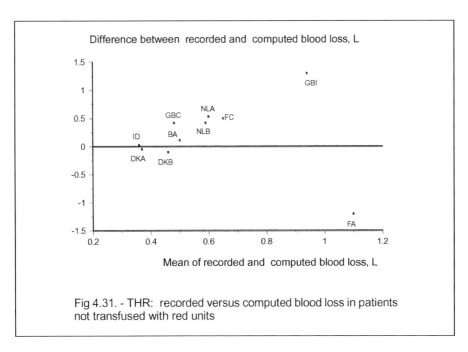

Fig 4.31. - THR: recorded versus computed blood loss in patients not transfused with red units

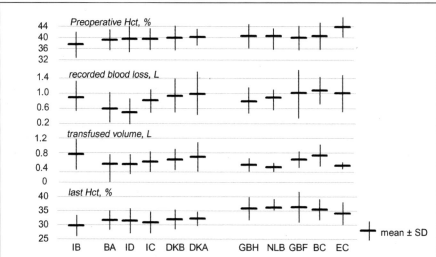

Fig 4.32. - THR: relationships among preoperative Hct, blood loss, transfused red cell volume and last Hct in patients transfused with red units. Only hospitals are reported where the mean difference between recorded and computed blood loss did not exceed 0.4 L. Transfused volumes paralleled blood loss volumes in the majority of the hospitals

Complications of blood transfusion

No overall frequency of transfusion complications (Table 4.9) could be estimated since the records were confined to so few hospitals.

Table 4.9. THR: complications of blood transfusion

	Hospital number	Type	Involved patients	Transfused patients
Allogeneic				
	2	haemolytic reaction	2	108
	3	skin reaction	5	171
	5	fever/rigors	11	224
	1	laboratory mismatch	1	53
reported in	7/31			
Autologous	1			
		fever/rigors	2	16
reported in	1/19			

Complications of surgery

Distributions of age, gender, preoperative Hct value, perioperative and postoperative blood loss were rather similar in the sub-set of reoperated patients and overall patient set, whereas the last Hct value was lower, and postsurgical LOS longer (Table 4.10). The median age of five patients

Table 4.10. THR: complications of surgery

	Hospital number	Patient number	Age, years[1]	Gender M:F	Preoperative Hct %[1]	Blood loss, L perioperative	postoperative	Red units per patient	Last Hct %[1]	Postoperative LOS days	Death: days after surgery[1]
Reoperation for bleeding	7/31	11	65 (46-86)	4:7	39 (35-44)	0.6 (0.2-1.2)	0.4 (0.1-1.0)	4 (1-8)	29 (27-33)	23 (7-47)	
recorded in		7/1 647 (5/11 in IC)			9/11	9/11	8/11		7/11		
deaths		5	70 (67-82)	2:3	· (38-46)	· (0.3-0.7)	· (0.3-1.1)	· (3-3)	· (28-34)		14 (1-58)
recorded in	4/31	5/1 647			4/5	4/5	3/5	4/5	3/5		

[1] Median (range).
· = not calculated due to the small sample size.

who died was higher than that of the overall patient set, while no remarkable differences were observed among the available data.

The median LOS before surgery was three days (hinges: 1-6) and after surgery 14 days (hinges: 12-18). The preoperative LOS was shorter in hospitals of central-northern Europe (Figure 4.33) than in those of the Mediterranean area (two (hinges: 1-3) versus six (hinges: 3-10) days, median values).

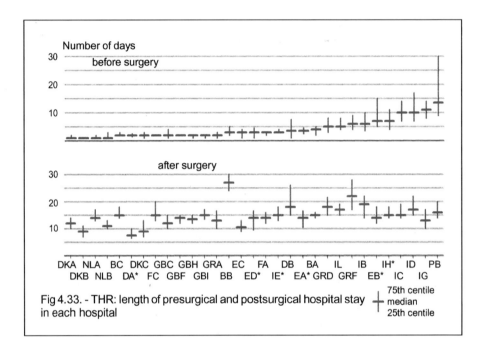

Fig 4.33. - THR: length of presurgical and postsurgical hospital stay in each hospital

75th centile
median
25th centile

VI. Costs

The overall costs due to product use were ECU 192 per operated patient. Of these, 86% was due to red units. The lowest and highest costs observed among hospitals were ECU 60 to 383 per patient operated (Figure 4.34).

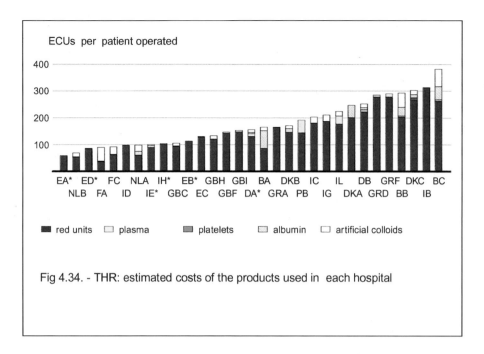

Fig 4.34. - THR: estimated costs of the products used in each hospital

VII. Comments on THR

THR patients received red units (81%), artificial colloids (49%), albumin (13%) and plasma (6%). These proportions, however, differed greatly among hospitals, even within a country: from 29 to 100% for red units, 0 to 98% for artificial colloids, 0 to 76% for albumin and 0 to 95% for plasma. Also, the median amount of product administered to recipients showed wide variations among hospitals: from two to five for red units; 0.5 to 2.5 L for artificial colloids, 9 to 41 g for albumin. In a few hospitals (BB, BC, IL), the wider the variety of the product used, the higher was the proportion of recipients and also the amount of product administered to patients.

Some variables were found to affect the proportion of patients perioperatively transfused with red units and the mean number of red units per recipient. These were: gender, preoperative Hct, blood loss and the high use of autotransfusion. However, interhospital differences persisted, even after adjustment for age, gender and perioperative blood loss. The size of this difference was greater than those due to the examined variables. This is confirmed by the different effect of the examined variables in different hospitals. Among them, the final value of Hct seemed to relate to transfusion use in some hospitals. In GRF, for instance, the highest values of the last Hct were found and were associated with the transfusion of all operated patients. In contrast, in FA, the lowest last Hct values observed in this study were associated with the lowest proportion of transfused patients. In addition, transfusions withheld perioperatively and administered only postoperatively also played a role in two hospitals (FC, BA).

The use of different surgical techniques (e.g. cemented, non-cemented or personalized prostheses) is a further, not studied co-factor that may account for differences in transfusion. If these procedural differences are important, however, differences in blood loss would be expected to suggest an effect.

The use of autotransfusion also varied among hospitals: the proportion of operated patients transfused with autologous red units varied from 0 to 100%. The use of autotransfusion sometimes had a number of drawbacks. Sufficient time was not allowed for PABD patients to regain their pre-donation Hct values, thus increasing their probability of being transfused. In one hospital (IB) a number of PABD patients received red units that had been set aside for the operation before this was actually performed, suggesting that clinicians did not accept the post-donation Hct value as adequate for operation. In a few other hospitals, PABD units were separated into red blood cell concentrates and fresh frozen plasma.

PABD patients were younger and in a high proportion male, features that made them appropriate candidates for donation. In other settings, these patients would have been candidates for not receiving transfusion. Perioperative transfusion was evidently rather independent of preoperative Hct value and blood loss in those hospitals with a high use of autotransfusion, suggesting that patients were at times transfused largely because autologous blood was available. These observations have to be interpreted with caution since the time during which the study was performed coincided with a period of enthusiastic promotion and acceptance of autotransfusion and anticipated the forthcoming availability of recombinant human erythropoietin. Autotransfusion was used in more hospitals in the Mediterranean area, probably in response to a desire to conserve resources of allogeneic red units and also to reduce risks of hepatitis transmission (it should be noted that the period of the study also preceded the routine implementation of donor screening for the hepatitis C virus).

The effect of some variables on the number of units per patient transfused was similar to that observed on the proportion of patients transfused, although the differences from hospital to hospital, after adjustment for age, gender, preoperative Hct and blood loss, were less striking. The number of units transfused per recipient was not related to preoperative Hct or to blood loss in hospitals with little or no autotransfusion, suggesting that there may be a 'standard dose' of red units. In contrast, in hospitals with a high use of autotransfusion, the use of IBS allowed retrieval of shed blood. Possibly, differences in volume of the red units could be one reason underlying the interhospital differences in the number of units transfused. Differences persisted, however, even when only hospitals not using autotransfusion (all of them from the same broad geographic area) were considered.

Among hospitals using little or no autotransfusion, a positive correlation was found between the proportion of patients transfused and the mean number of units per patient transfused, indicating that in hospitals where more patients were transfused, each patient was given more units. The correlation was not found in the remaining surgical procedures studied; there, however, the set of hospitals was different.

The threshold for postoperative transfusion of red units was a mean Hct value of 26% ± 3.

Comparison with the literature is not easy, due to the lack of standard measures used among various authors to express blood use, differences in the number of hospitals and patients surveyed in various studies, in the year of the study and in the location of the hospitals. However, after standardizing some published data, comparison shows that the majority of the Sanguis hospitals fell within the wide range of variability seen in other studies, [4-5] with about one third of the Sanguis hospitals located above the upper published data.

Nearly two thirds of patients receiving allogeneic plasma were also transfused with red units during the same 24-hour period, effectively reconstituting whole blood. In one hospital (PB), nearly all operated patients were transfused with both red units and liquid plasma. This practice negates the widely accepted concept of blood component therapy and unnecessarily increases patient risk. In another hospital (GRF), about one third of the patients received plasma even though 69% of the transfused red units were whole blood. In hospital IL, two thirds of patients received autologous plasma. Furthermore, 75% of all plasma recipients were given only one or two units, doses usually considered to be ineffective in the treatment of coagulation disorders.

Hospitals differed in the use of colloids according to a geographic pattern: the proportion of albumin recipients was three times higher in the hospitals of central-northern Europe than in those of the Mediterranean area, and that of artificial colloids 68 times higher. In this case, diversities may be largely explained by a different availability of products. However, variations from hospital to hospital were observed in both the proportion of recipients and amount given per recipient, even within one country. In some hospitals dextrans might have been used to help prevent the occurrence of DVT, although this was not reported in the clinical record. Diversities persisted, however, even when hospitals using dextrans are not considered. Although in THR the need to replace extracellular fluid losses is moderate, compared for example with intra-abdominal procedures, in some hospitals the proportion of THR patients given colloids was comparable to that for COLE patients in other hospitals. Clinical preferences, therefore, seem to be the most likely explanation for variation. The fact that the choice of fluid for the management of acute hypovolaemia remains controversial and unsupported by proof of superior efficacy of any type of product, [16-21] probably adds to the general confusion that pervades this area of treatment.

Variability was observed not only in the use of the studied products. Administration of anticoagulants for the prevention of DVT, and the preoperative LOS, also varied widely.

Recorded blood loss volumes, besides being infrequently recorded, are known to be rather inaccurate and subjective. However, it was decided to consider them when they were available for the majority of patients, on the assumption that this information would be part of the decision process to transfuse a given patient (as in fact the analysis demonstrated). Furthermore, a comparison between recorded and computed blood loss volumes showed that, while they were similar in some hospitals, overestimates of blood loss were probably made in a majority of hospitals and underestimates in a minority. [22]

5.0. Coronary artery bypass graft (CABG)

Surgical revascularization of ischaemic heart is currently a cornerstone of treatment for patients with ischaemic heart disease. Surgical mortality varies with patient risk factors, such as acuity of symptoms and state of ventricular function. Mortality rate in the multivessel younger age patient group with good left ventricular function is about 1%; in acute ischaemic syndromes requiring urgent surgery, operative mortality may vary from 2 to 25%. The effect of age is to double the operative mortality in patients over 70, especially in those who have had ischaemic events. Obstructed coronary artery vessel(s) are bypassed with the use of either internal mammary artery (superior long-term patency) or reversed segments of the saphenous vein, more rarely of the gastro-epiploic.

Case report forms were available from 1 166 patients in 21 hospitals and nine countries: 818 (70%) in 13 hospitals in six central-northern European countries and 348 (30%) in eight hospitals in three Mediterranean countries (Figure 5.1).

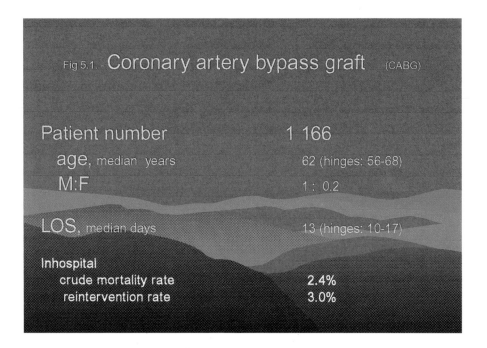

Fig 5.1. - Coronary artery bypass graft (CABG)

Patient number	1 166
age, median years	62 (hinges: 56-68)
M:F	1 : 0.2
LOS, median days	13 (hinges: 10-17)
Inhospital	
crude mortality rate	2.4%
reintervention rate	3.0%

I. Patient data and some variables related to surgery

Table 5.1 reports, by hospital, the number, age and gender of patients, and the values of some variables related to surgery. Among hospitals, the median age ranged from 58 to 66 years, although a median value of 60 to 65 years was observed in the majority of them. The M:F ratio ranged from 3:1 to 25:1.

135

Table 5.1. CABG: patient data and some variables related to surgery

	PA	ED*	IG	DKC	DKA	EC	EA*	GBG	PB	NLA	FC	DB	FB	GBF	ID	BA	BB	BC	DA	GBA	IH
Patient number	70	1	26	62	60	58	11	72	43	62	30	34	63	72	84	75	78	67	71	72	55
Age (years), median value	62	•	63	60	58	62	71	61	58	66	63	61	64	58	62	64	64	62	63	61	58
range	37-80		47-76	41-75	40-75	35-92	47-76	44-79	33-71	49-90	37-80	37-75	38-84	37-80	40-78	38-82	40-77	43-76	44-79	41-75	37-75
M:F ratio	4.8		25	4.2	3.6	6.2	1.7	7.0	7.6	4.6	6.5	4.7	9.5	4.1	4.6	4.3	4.6	7.4	4.5	3.0	8.2
Preoperative Hct																					
% Po with	17		65	92	95	81	100	94	100	95	90	91	95	87	77	97	100	100	90	96	80
%, median value	41		42	43	42	41	39	42	45	43	42	44	40	43	41	42	40	41	42	44	40
range	37-48		36-49	37-50	20-54	33-50	32-47	33-50	38-54	32-50	35-48	33-47	30-46	33-52	30-49	30-49	28-48	32-51	31-52	37-53	32-52
Drugs % Po		•																			
anticoagulant only	100			77	43	48	91	100	77	100	73	3	36	96	100	96	100	6	58	97	89
haemostatic + anticoagulant			100	3		52			33			97	64			4		94	42	1	11
Graft % Po		•																			
saphenous			19.2	14.5	51.7	41.4	63.6	11.1	62.8	14.5	3.3	47.0	4.8	15.3	29.8	10.7	21.8	79.1	45.1	43.1	7.3
mammary			80.8	16.1	20.0	8.6	27.3	1.4	2.3	27.4	43.3	5.9	11.1	1.4	14.3	21.3	15.4	1.5	7.0	6.9	5.4
mammary and saphenous	100			69.4	28.3	50.0	9.1	83.3	34.9	58.1	53.3	47.1	84.1	83.3	55.9	68.0	62.8	19.4	47.9	50.0	87.3
Duration of surgery		•																			
% Po with	83			98	52	98	100	67	100	58			75	65	62	76	77	79		78	100
median minutes	155			205	200	280	200	240	300	180			270	210	72	300	240	240		192	360
range	140-180			100-315	80-290	200-440	150-300	110-360	180-420	22-300			120-450	135-370	42-152	170-480	120-360	130-450		105-640	240-720
Blood loss																					
perioperative		•																			
% Po with	81		100	97	8	90	27			81	60	3	3			3	100	92	10		
median L	0.75		0.50	0.65	•	0.90	•			0.34	0.62	•	•			•	0.49	0.36	•		
range	0.1-2.9		0.25-1.7	0.2-3.0	•	0.4-3.1	•			0.05-1.3	0.07-2.3	•	•			•	0.11-1.2	0.1-2.0	•		
postoperative		•																			
% Po with	17		100	2	5	95	54	15		34	40	71	19	97	99	99	99	95	69	100	100
median L	0.8		0.4	•	•	0.4	•	1.3		0.8	0.5	0.6	1.1	0.7	0.4	0.9	0.8	0.6	0.5	1.0	0.5
range	0.3-2.0		0.1-1.0	•	•	0.0-1.0	•	0.5-2.3		0.0-1.4	0.2-1.5	0.2-1.2	0.3-10.8	0.3-2.2	0.1-1.3	0.3-4.3	0.3-3.4	0.2-2.8	0.2-3.0	0.2-13.1	0.2-4.2

Po = patients operated.
Anaesthesia: all patients had general anaesthesia, except 8% of patients operated in GBF.
Hospital code and * = less than 20 patients.
• = not calculated due to the small sample size.

The median preoperative Hct value was 42% (hinges: 39-44%) and in all hospitals it was higher than 40%.

General anaesthesia was used in 99.5% and combined anaesthesia in 0.5% of patients (GBF).

95% of patients received a drug acting on the coagulation system. 74% of patients received an anticoagulant drug and 21% also a haemostatic drug. Figure 5.2 shows the percentage of recipients according to the time of administration in respect to the day of surgery: 5% of patients appeared not to have received a drug; this, however, should probably be interpreted as a non-record, since systemic anticoagulation treatment during extracorporeal circulation is universal.

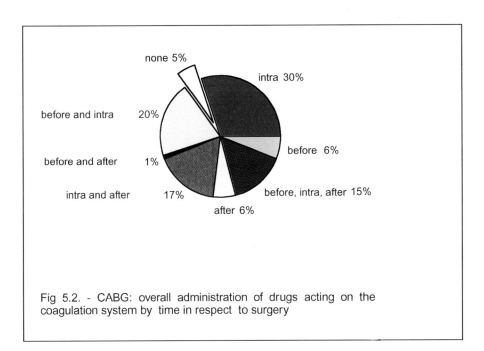

Fig 5.2. - CABG: overall administration of drugs acting on the coagulation system by time in respect to surgery

Figure 5.3 illustrates the distribution of the type of drug administered before, during and after surgery. Figure 5.4 shows the variations among hospitals in the distribution of the time of drug administration.

60% of patients underwent a mammary artery and saphenous vein grafts, 27% a saphenous vein graft only, and 13% a mammary artery graft only. Mammary and saphenous grafts predominated in 13 hospitals, mammary graft in one, and saphenous graft in three hospitals. Mammary with gastroepiploic grafts were used in 1% of patients.

Information on duration of surgery was available in 66% of patients. In 16 hospitals, the information was available in more than 50% of patients. The median recorded duration was 230 minutes (hinges: 180-300). The lowest and highest median values were 72 and 360 minutes.

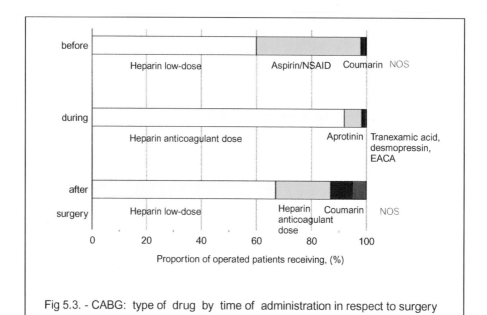

Fig 5.3. - CABG: type of drug by time of administration in respect to surgery

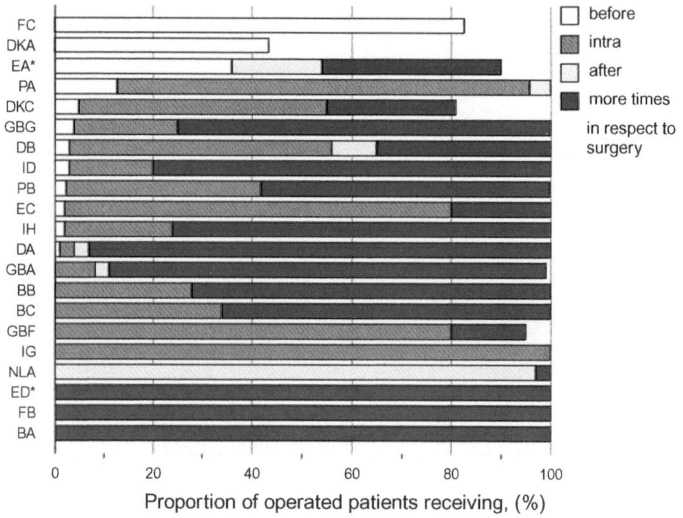

Fig 5.4. - CABG: administration of drugs acting on the coagulation system by time in respect to surgery in each hospital

Perioperative blood loss was documented in 36% of patients and postoperative loss in 67%. The median volume was 0.6 L (hinges: 0.4-0.9) for perioperative and 0.7 L (hinges: 0.4-1.0) for postoperative blood loss. Figure 5.5 shows the cumulative distribution of perioperative blood loss volumes. The lowest values seem likely to reflect underestimates of loss.

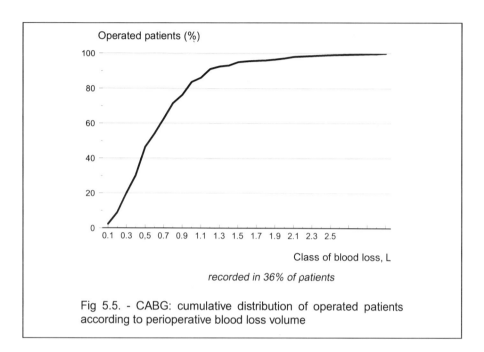

Fig 5.5. - CABG: cumulative distribution of operated patients according to perioperative blood loss volume

II. Transfusion data

The distribution of hospitals according to the type of products used (Table 5.2) showed groups of three hospitals using: only blood components, blood components and albumin, blood components and artificial colloids, while 12 hospitals used all three types of product.

Hospitals of half of the countries (B, D, F, DK) used the same types of product.

II.1.0. *Red units*

Of operated patients, 88% were transfused with 4 339 red units, the percentage of patients receiving red units varying among hospitals from 17 to 100. No difference was observed in the proportion of patients transfused in hospitals of central-northern Europe compared to that of the Mediterranean area.

In transfused patients, the median number of red units transfused was four (hinges: 2-5) and differed among hospitals from one to five. Of operated patients, 31% received a number of red units higher than four (Figure 5.6).

Table 5.2. CABG: transfusion data

	PA	ED*	IG	DKC	DKA	EC	EA*	GBG	PB	NLA	FC	DB	FB	GBF	ID	BA	BB	BC	DA	GBA	IH
Red units	–	–	–	–	–	–	–	–	–	–	–	–	–	–	–	–	–	–	–	–	–
patients transfused/operated (%)	17.1	100	100	72.6	96.7	100	54.5	95.8	100	59.7	80	85.3	88.9	88.9	94	98.7	98.7	100	100	100	100
units per transfused patient median	1	•	4	3	4	4	2	3	5	2	3.5	3	2.5	2	2	5	4	5	5	4	4
hinges	1-2.5		3-5	1-5	3-5	3-5	2-4	2-4	4-6	2-3	3-6.5	2-4	1-4	1-3	2-2	4-7	2.5-5	4-7	4-8	3-5	2-6
Plasma																					
patients transfused/operated (%)	1.4		34.6	33.9	95	37.9	9.1	27.8	100	66.1	13.3	5.9	85.7	12.5	19	12	47.4	16.4	70.4	15.3	67.3
units per transfused patient median	•		1	4	10	3	•	2	4	4	2.5	•	2	6	4	4	2	2	3	2	4
hinges			1-1	2-4	8-13	2-4		2-4	3-6	2-6	1.5-4.5		1-4	6-6	3-4	2-4	1-2	2-4	2-4	2-3	3-7
Platelets																					
patients transfused/operated (%)				11.3	38.3		9.1	22.2	9.3	3.2	3.3	2.9	3.2	4.2	42.9	4	0.1	1.5	2.8	15.3	21.8
units per transfused patient median				4	4		•	5	•	•	•	•	•	•		•				5	8.5
hinges				2-6	3-6			4.5-5												5-25	7-10
Cryoprecipitate																					
patients transfused/operated (%)					1.7				2.3	4.8				2.8					4.2		
Albumin																					
patients administered/operated (%)				11.3	55	10.3				45.2	46.7	76.5	74.6	75	42.9	89.3	92.3	97	87.3	87.5	100
grams per recipient median				21	38	nos				41	61.5	95	42	226	21	62	61	92	52	81	89
hinges				13-41	13-67					21-41	42-63	64-115	41-84	113-338	11-22	41-83	41-82	71-112	38-77	61-102	51-121
Colloids																					
patients administered/operated (%)							54.5	87.5	95.3	72.6	100	67.6	28.6	48.6	2.4	98.7	93.5	76.1	95.8	31.9	5.4
L per recipient median							2	1	2	0.5	1.5	1	1	0.5	•	4	1.4	0.7	1.5	0.5	•
hinges							1.0-2.5	0.5-1.5	1.0-2.5	0.5-1.0	0.75-2.0	0.5-1.0	0.5-1.0	0.5-1.0		3.0-5.0	1.0-1.7	0.4-1.0	1.2-2.0	0.5-2.0	
Patients for whom the number of autologous blood units was not known										1.6			44.4	47.2			2.6	7.5		11.1	

Hospitals are aggregated according to products used.
• = quantities not calculated due to the small sample size.
Hospital code and * = less than 20 patients.
[1] Use of autotransfusion.
nos = not otherwise specified.

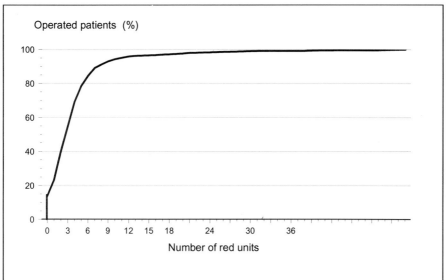

Fig 5.6. - CABG: cumulative distribution of operated patients according to the number of red units transfused

II.1.1. *Allogeneic and autologous transfusion*

Globally, 439 patients were transfused with 1 800 allogeneic red units, 170 with 386 autologous red units, and 414 with 1 404 allogeneic and 749 autologous red units (Figure 5.7). In 4.7% of operated patients, information on the number of the units transfused (autologous in the great majority of cases) was incomplete.

Wide interhospital variations in both the percentage of patients transfused with autologous and/or allogeneic units and the number of autologous and allogeneic units per patient operated were observed (Figure 5.8). In hospitals of the central-northern European area, the proportion of patients transfused with autologous units was half that observed in the Mediterranean area (RR = 0.5 (0.5 to 0.6)).

IBS, alone or associated with other techniques, was the autotransfusion technique most widely used (Figure 5.9). The intraoperatively salvaged units were double those provided by PABD or PIH (Figure 5.7).

Figure 5.10 shows a comparison of red unit use between the Sanguis data and those of multicentre studies available in the literature.

II.1.2. *Allogeneic whole blood use*

Of all transfused red units, 11% were whole blood. 16, 25, 30 and 91% of the red units transfused in four hospitals (GBG, BC, BA, GBF) were whole blood (Figure 5.11).

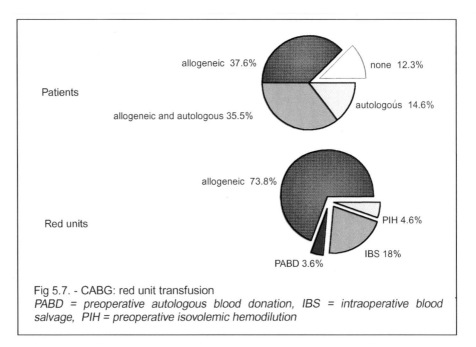

Fig 5.7. - CABG: red unit transfusion
PABD = preoperative autologous blood donation, IBS = intraoperative blood salvage, PIH = preoperative isovolemic hemodilution

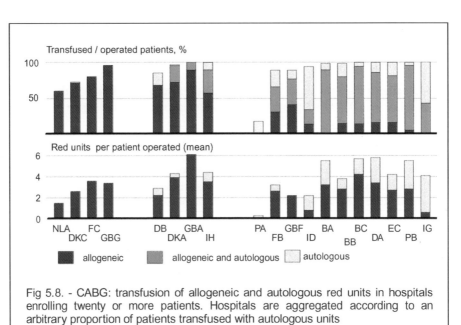

Fig 5.8. - CABG: transfusion of allogeneic and autologous red units in hospitals enrolling twenty or more patients. Hospitals are aggregated according to an arbitrary proportion of patients transfused with autologous units

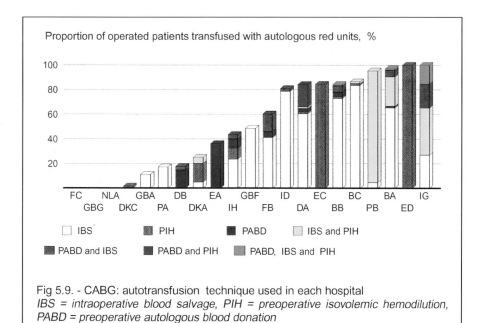

Fig 5.9. - CABG: autotransfusion technique used in each hospital
*IBS = intraoperative blood salvage, PIH = preoperative isovolemic hemodilution,
PABD = preoperative autologous blood donation*

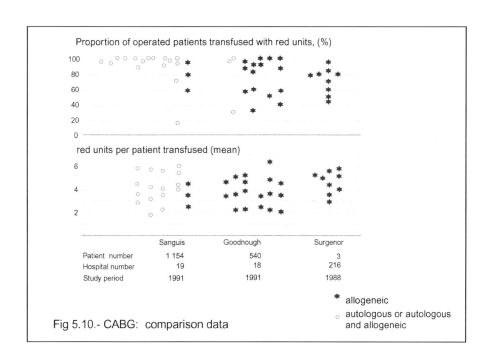

Fig 5.10.- CABG: comparison data

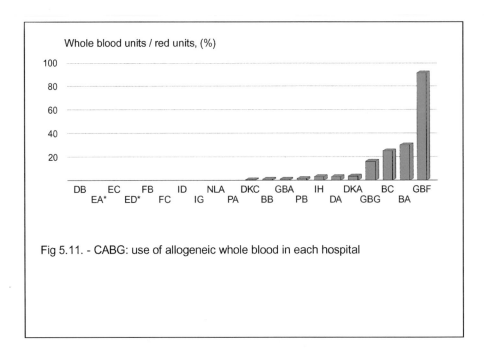

Whole blood units / red units, (%)

Fig 5.11. - CABG: use of allogeneic whole blood in each hospital

II.1.3. *Time of transfusion*

As shown in Figure 5.12 almost all transfusions occurred during the perioperative period. Postoperative transfusions involved only a small proportion of patients with the exception of hospital FC in which about one quarter of patients were transfused postoperatively (Figure 5.13).

II.2.0. *Platelets*

In all 624 platelet concentrates were transfused to 90 patients (8%) in 16 of 21 hospitals, 13 of them located in central-northern Europe (Figure 5.14).

The median number of units of platelets per recipient was five (hinges: 3-8).

In two hospitals (BA, BC) only apheresis platelets were used, accounting for 2% of the total.

II.3.0. *Plasma*

2 152 plasma units were transfused to 454 (39%) patients. Plasma was used, although in very different proportions of patients, in all hospitals except ED. More than two thirds of the plasma recipients and more than three quarters of plasma units were transfused in a minority of hospitals (DA, DKA, FB, IH, NLA, PB) (Figure 5.15). The percentage of patients receiving plasma in the hospitals of central-northern Europe was twice that of hospitals in the Mediterranean area (RR = 2 (1 to 2)). The median number of units given to plasma recipients was four (hinges: 2-6).

144

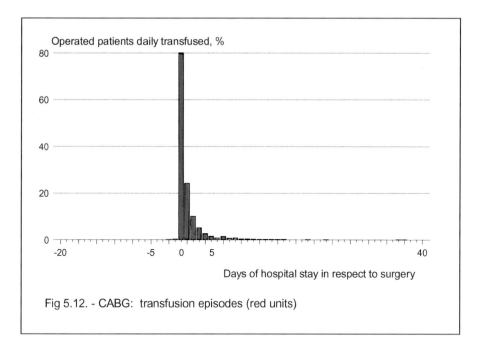

Fig 5.12. - CABG: transfusion episodes (red units)

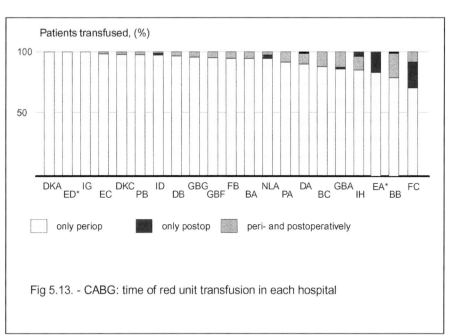

Fig 5.13. - CABG: time of red unit transfusion in each hospital

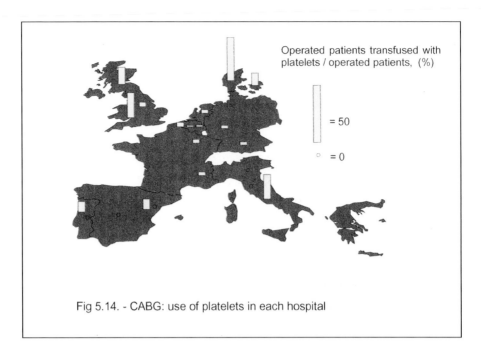

Fig 5.14. - CABG: use of platelets in each hospital

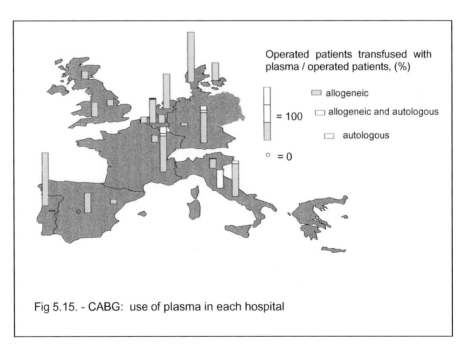

Fig 5.15. - CABG: use of plasma in each hospital

In all 127 (5.9%) plasma units were autologous (Figures 5.15 and 5.16) and were used in a few hospitals, one of them (FB) accounting for 4%; 1 089 (50.6%) were liquid plasma (EA, EC, NLA, PB, DKA, the latter alone accounting for 28%), 899 (41.8%) were fresh frozen plasma, and 37 (1.7%) were collected by apheresis (BA and BC accounting for 35 of the 37 units).

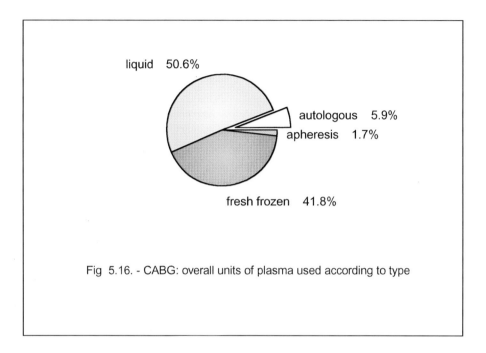

Fig 5.16. - CABG: overall units of plasma used according to type

Of 430 patients receiving allogeneic plasma, 376 were also given red cell concentrates, 349 during the same 24-hour period.

II.4.0. *Cryoprecipitate*

In all 107 units of cryoprecipitate were given to 10 patients in five hospitals, four of them located in central-northern Europe. Of the units, 65% were in one hospital (GBA). The median number of units was nine (hinges: 2-20).

II.5.0. *Albumin*

In all 57 580 g of albumin was administered to 635 (54%) patients in 15 of 21 hospitals, 12 of them being located in central-northern Europe, where the percentage of recipients was twice that in hospitals of the Mediterranean area (RR = 2 (2 to 3)). In recipients, a median of 64 g (hinges: 41-103) was administered (Figure 5.17).

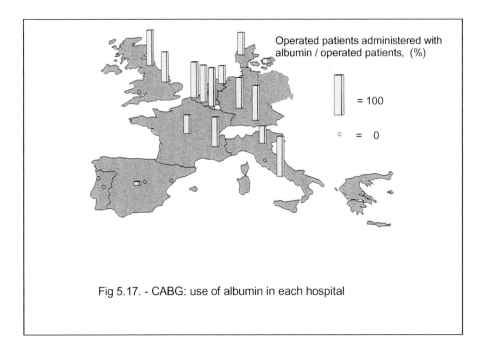

Operated patients administered with albumin / operated patients, (%)

= 100

° = 0

Fig 5.17. - CABG: use of albumin in each hospital

Hospitals using albumin differed widely in both the percentage of recipients (10 to 100%) and in the amount given per recipient (range of the medians was 21 to 226 g). A high use of albumin was observed in a few hospitals (GBF accounting for 26% and the three Belgian hospitals for 27% of the total amount used).

II.6.0. *Artificial colloids*

In all 944 L of artificial colloids were administered to 555 patients (48%) in 15 of 21 hospitals (Figure 5.18). In recipients the median volume was 1.0 L (hinges: 0.5-2.0). The proportion of recipients and the volume per recipient varied even among hospitals using colloids, from 2 to 100% and from 0.5 to 4.0 L. 38% of the recipients and 53% of the volume used were in three hospitals (BA, BB, DA). Consequently, the percentage of patients given artificial colloids in hospitals of central-northern Europe was five times (Figure 5.18) that observed in the Mediterranean area (RR = 5 (4 to 6)).

Of all artificial colloid used, 84% was gelatin, 15% HES and 1% dextran. The volumes of each colloid per operated patient in each hospital are reported in Figure 5.19.

The median volume was 0.5 L (hinges: 0.5-1.0) for HES, 0.75 L (hinges: 0.5-1.0) for dextran, and 1.5 L (hinges: 0.75-2.5) for gelatin. Hospitals differed mainly in the use of the latter colloid, the median volume per recipient ranging from 0.5 to 4.0 L.

The variety of clinical use of products in the hospitals is shown in Figure 5.20 and that in hospitals grouped according to country in Figure 5.21.

148

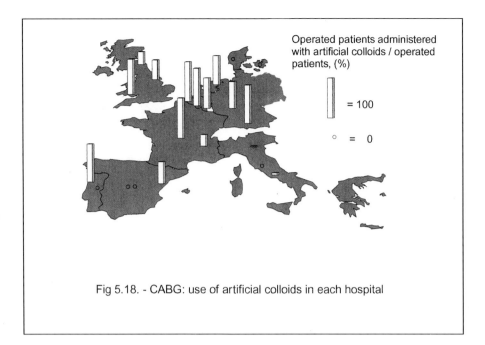

Fig 5.18. - CABG: use of artificial colloids in each hospital

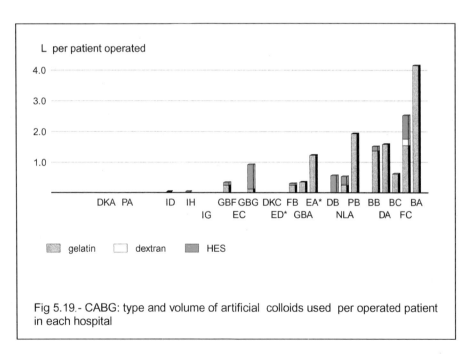

Fig 5.19.- CABG: type and volume of artificial colloids used per operated patient in each hospital

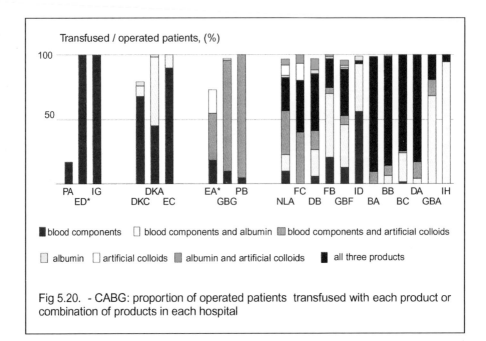

Fig 5.20. - CABG: proportion of operated patients transfused with each product or combination of products in each hospital

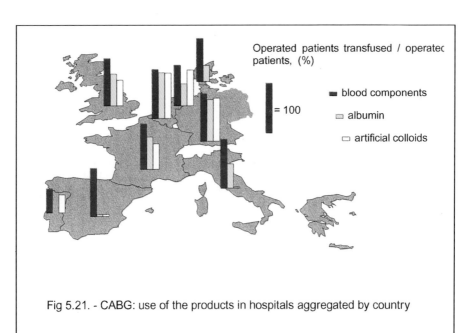

Fig 5.21. - CABG: use of the products in hospitals aggregated by country

III. Reasons for perioperative transfusion documented in the medical record

III.1. *Red units*

A reason was found in 17% of transfused patients (Figure 5.22.) in 15 of 21 hospitals, most of them from central-northern Europe. Reasons given were a low Hct value (9%), bleeding (6%) and others (2%).

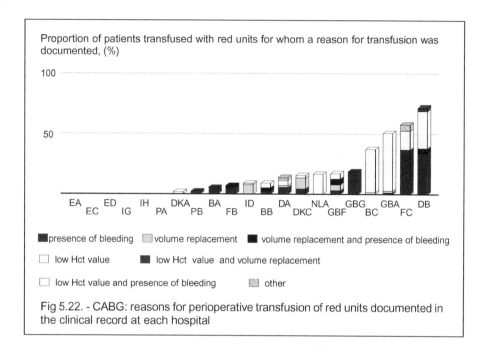

Fig 5.22. - CABG: reasons for perioperative transfusion of red units documented in the clinical record at each hospital

III.2. *Plasma*

Reasons were given in 23% of the recipients in 13 hospitals. A PT value was found in 71 patients (16%), half of them from Belgian hospitals, and volume replacement in 3% of recipients.

III.3. *Platelets*

In 32% of platelet recipients a reason, usually bleeding, was recorded for transfusion. In 7% of the recipients a platelet count was recorded which ranged from 36 to $88 \times 10^9/L$.

III.4. *Albumin*

Reasons were found in 14% of the recipients of 10 hospitals; in nearly all patients they were represented by volume replacement.

III.5. *Artificial colloids*

Reasons were found in 33% of patients and in eight hospitals. Volume replacement was the given reason in the great majority of cases.

IV. Variables associated with red unit transfusion

IV.1. *Transfused versus untransfused patients*

The variables (Table 5.3) under study were rather similar in both the sub-sets of transfused and untransfused patients. Of untransfused patients, 49% were from one hospital (PA).

IV.2. *Preoperative transfusion of red units*

Of five patients (0.4% operated), three received their own pre-donated units before operation. Patients preoperatively transfused in four hospitals were three males and two females, aged 53 to 65 years (range). The only Hct available was that recorded the day of transfusion and it ranged from 28 to 38%, median 33%.

IV.3. *Perioperative transfusion of patients with red units*

Indicator: proportion of operated patients perioperatively transfused with red units (mean percentage ± SE)

Hospitals: six (31%) of 19 enrolling 20 or more patients

Patients: 254 (26%) of 961, after exclusion of females (due to the small sample size), deaths and reinterventions

Variables: age, preintervention Hct, type of graft (saphenous vein only versus mammary artery, alone or with saphenous vein), blood loss

Since the effect of a variable on the probability of a patient being transfused cannot be studied when all or nearly all patients (90% or more) are transfused, two thirds of the hospitals showing this feature were not analysed. A comparison between patients of hospitals included and not included in the analysis, however, showed no systematic difference in the proportion of patients aged more than 65 years, the proportion of patients with a preoperative Hct value lower than 41%, whereas the proportion of autotransfused patients was higher in the hospitals not included in the analysis. A special case was represented by hospital PB, where all operated patients were transfused, although they were younger and had higher preoperative (and last) Hct values than patients of all the remaining hospitals.

On average, the probability of an operated patient being transfused (Part I, Figure 0.14) increased with increasing age (difference between the highest and lowest age class = +15%), with an increasing blood loss volume (difference between the highest and lowest class of blood loss = +10%), and decreased with increasing preoperative Hct values (difference between the highest and lowest class of Hct = −38%). Those patients with a mammary artery graft, alone or with other grafts, had a lower probability of being transfused compared to those with only a saphenous graft (71% ±1.5 versus 92% ±2.0). This finding has not been further explored.

Table 5.3. CABG: comparison between patients transfused and not transfused with red units during the hospital stay

	Patients transfused			Patients not transfused	95% confidence interval of the difference[2]
	allogeneic	allogeneic and autologous	autologous		
Patient number	439	414	170	143	
Age,[1] years	62 (56-68)	63 (57-68)	60 (52-66)	62 (52-68)	−0.7 to 0.7
M:F	*3.8*	4.7	14.2	*7.5*	*2 to 15*
Hct preoperatively[1] %	*42 (39-44)*	41 (39-44)	42 (39-44)	*44 (42-45)*	*1.1 to 2.9*
Percentage of patients with	93	92	84	61	
Anaesthesia, regional and/or combined, % Po	0.7	0.5		0.6	
Anticoagulants, % Po	91	98	100	94	
Haemostatic, % Po	14	29.7	28	10	
Duration of surgery,[1] minutes	225 (180-280)	260 (215-302)	190 (80-260)	160 (150-200)	
Percentage of patients with	66	68	50	78	
Blood loss, L[1]					
perioperative	0.6 (0.4-0.9)	0.6 (0.4-0.8)	0.5 (0.4-0.8)	0.6 (0.3-1.0)	0.8 to 1.2[3]
Percentage of patients with	28	36	30	64	
total	1.3 (1.0-1.6)	1.2 (0.9-1.6)	1.0 (0.8-1.3)	1.1 (0.9-1.6)	
Percentage of patients with	11	36	30	9.3	
Percent of patients transfused with					
plasma	45.6	46.4	21.7		
albumin	54.2	69.3	43.4	27.3	
artificial colloids	45.6	65.0	27.6	27.3	
PABD, percent patients		87	100		
Stated reason for transfusion, % Pt	25	13	4		
Reintervention for bleeding, % Po	5.47	2.42	0.66		
In-hospital crude mortality rate, % Po	2.73	3.38		1.2	
Last Hct,[1] %	34 (32-37)	34 (31-37)	32 (30-34)	'33 (30-36)	
Percentage of patients with	97	99	99	64	
Hospital stay,[1] days	12 (9-16)	15 (12-20)	14 (11-19)	10 (8-15)	
before surgery	3 (2-5)	4 (2-7)	4 (2-7)	2 (1-4)	
after surgery	9 (7-11)	10 (9-13)	10 (9-12)	8 (7-10)	

Po = patients operated.
Pt = patients transfused.
[1] Median (hinges).
[2] Between patients not transfused and transfused with allogeneic red units, after exclusion of deaths and reinterventions.
[3] Performed on ln values.
Note: *significant differences are shown in bold italics.*

Hospitals with a large use of autotransfusion showed a probability of patient transfusion higher than those with low autotransfusion use (86% ± 0.9 versus 67% ± 0.5, difference = 19%). This finding was observed even when preoperative Hct values were over 44% (66% ± 1.9 versus 47% ± 1.5, difference = 19%).

In ascending order, differences in the proportion of patients transfused attributable to blood loss were 10%, to age 15%, to type of graft 21% and to preoperative Hct 38%.

Age affected patient transfusion in five of six hospitals, preoperative Hct in five of five hospitals (Figure 5.23) and blood loss in three of three hospitals (and was contradictory in one case) (Figure 5.24).

A summary of the effect of the studied variables within hospitals is given in Figure 5.25.

After adjustment for the effect of age and preoperative Hct values, the proportion of patients transfused still differed significantly among hospitals (Figure 5.26), i.e. from 62% ± 1.0 to 89% ± 1.3 (difference between the lowest and highest value accounting for 18%). Further adjustment also for blood loss was feasible in only two hospitals (NLA, DKC) where the values were 52% ± 0.7 and 63% ± 0.8 (difference between the highest and lowest value accounting for 9%).

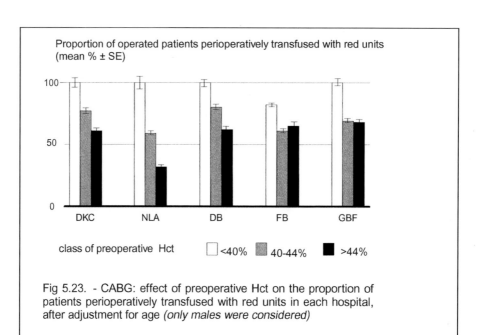

Fig 5.23. - CABG: effect of preoperative Hct on the proportion of patients perioperatively transfused with red units in each hospital, after adjustment for age (only males were considered)

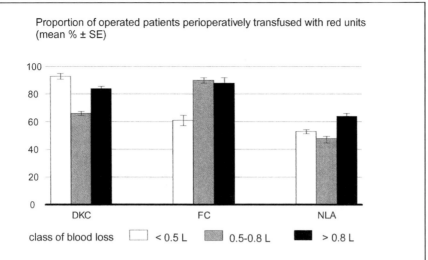

Proportion of operated patients perioperatively transfused with red units
(mean % ± SE)

class of blood loss ☐ < 0.5 L   ▨ 0.5-0.8 L   ■ > 0.8 L

Fig 5.24. - CABG: effect of blood loss on the proportion of operated
patients perioperatively transfused with red units, after adjustment for
age *(only males were considered)*

	age, yrs	graft	presurgery Hct, %	blood loss, L
	>61 vs <61	S vs M	>44 vs <40	>0.8 vs<0.5
hospital				
DB	⬆	⬆	⬇	/
DKC	⬆	⬆	⬇	⬇
FB	⬆	⬆	⬇	/
FC	⬆	⬆	?	⬆
GBF			⬇	/
NLA	⬆	⬆	⬇	⬆

⬆ increase   ⬇ decrease   blank = no variation   ? = poor sample size   / = data not available

Fig 5.25. - CABG: effect of some variables on the proportion of patients
perioperatively transfused with red units in each hospital, after adjustment for age. S =
saphenous vein graft, M= mammary artery graft *(only males were considered)*

155

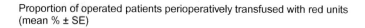

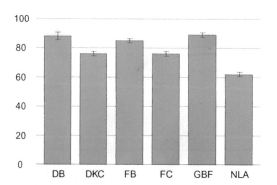

Proportion of operated patients perioperatively transfused with red units
(mean % ± SE)

Fig 5.26. - CABG: probability of a patient being perioperatively
transfused with red units in each hospital, after adjustment for age,
and preoperative Hct *(only males were considered)*

IV.4. *Perioperative transfusion of red units*

Indicator: red units per patient perioperatively transfused (mean number ± SE)

Hospitals: 18 (95%) of 19 enrolling 20 or more patients

Patients: 482 (50%) of 961, after exclusion of females (due to the small sample size), reoperations and deaths

Factors: age, preintervention Hct, graft and blood loss

On average, the higher the blood loss, the higher was the number of units transfused (difference between the highest and lowest class of blood loss = + 1.9), whereas the higher the preoperative Hct value, the slightly lower was the number of units transfused (difference between the highest and lowest class of preoperative Hct = − 0.6 unit). The number of units transfused was negligibly affected by age (3.6 versus 3.9 units per patient aged respectively less than 61 and over 65 years), and by type of graft (3.9 ± 0.07 in saphenous vein graft versus 3.8 ± 0.03 in mammary artery graft).

The number of units transfused in hospitals with a high use of autotransfusion was higher than in those with no/low autotransfusion use (4.1 ± 0.11 versus 3.1 ± 0.06). This finding was observed even at preoperative Hct values > 40% (4.3 ± 0.07 versus 2.9 ± 0.09) or at blood loss volumes < 0.5 L (3.2 ± 0.17 versus 2.5 ± 0.06).

Age affected the number of units transfused in five of 18 hospitals (not shown), preoperative Hct in 12 of 17 hospitals (Figure 5.27), but in two cases opposite to overall findings, and blood loss in three of six hospitals (Figure 5.28).

156

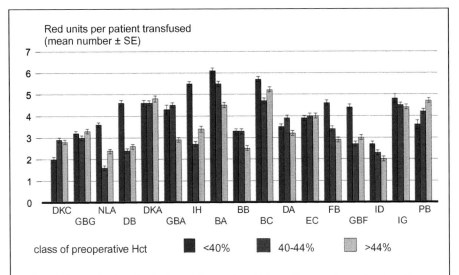

Fig 5.27. - CABG: effect of preintervention Hct on the number of red units per patient perioperatively transfused with red units in each hospital, after adjustment for age *(only males were considered)*

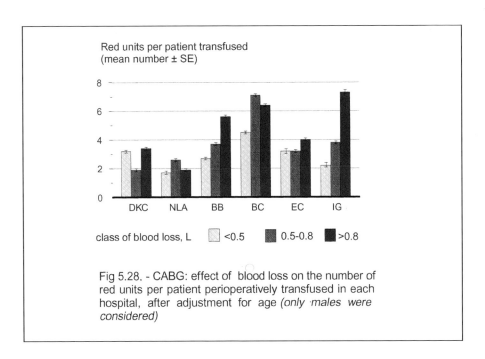

Fig 5.28. - CABG: effect of blood loss on the number of red units per patient perioperatively transfused in each hospital, after adjustment for age *(only males were considered)*

157

After adjustment for age and preoperative Hct, the mean number of units per patient transfused still varied among hospitals from 2.2 ± 0.1 to 5.3 ± 0.1 (difference = 3.1 units) (Figure 5.29). Further adjustment also for blood loss left major differences, i.e. from 3.4 ± 0.2 to 6.2 ± 0.2 units (difference = 2.8 units).

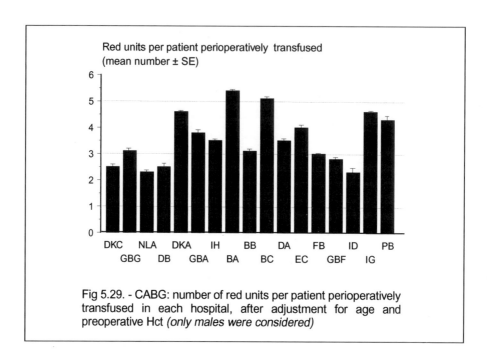

Red units per patient perioperatively transfused (mean number ± SE)

Fig 5.29. - CABG: number of red units per patient perioperatively transfused in each hospital, after adjustment for age and preoperative Hct *(only males were considered)*

In ascending order, the differences in the number of units per patient transfused attributable to preoperative Hct were 0.6 unit, to autotransfusion 1 unit, to blood loss 1.9 units and to other unknown, variables 2.8 units.

Postoperative transfusion of patients with red units

Profiles of transfused and untransfused patients, after exclusion of reinterventions and deaths, are shown in Table 5.4. The characteristic distinguishing the sub-set of transfused patients was the higher postoperative blood loss volume. On average, the threshold for transfusion occurred at an Hct value of 28% ± 2.9 to reach a postoperative one of 33% ± 3.3. The three Belgian hospitals accounted for 40% of all the patients transfused postoperatively.

Table 5.4. CABG: profiles of patients transfused and not transfused with red units in the postoperative period,[1] after exclusion of deaths and reoperated patients

	Patients transfused	Patients not transfused	95% confidence interval of the difference
Patient number	63	1 046	
Age, years[2]	63 ± 8.2	61 ± 9.3	−4.3 to 0.3
Percentage of males	87	84	−5 to −1
Hct pretransfusion, %[2]	28 ± 2.9		
Percentage of patients with	54		
Postoperative blood loss,[2] mL	*6.7 ± 0.6*	*6.5 ± 0.6*	*0.7 to 1.0*[3]
Percentage of patients with	86	66	
Units per patient transfused[2]	2.1 ± 1.0		
Last Hct, %[2]	33 ± 3.3	34 ± 4.1	2.4 to −0.6
Percentage of patients with	48	93	
Postsurgical LOS, days[2]	15.8 ± 9	10.4 ± 5.8	

[1] From the fourth day after surgery to discharge.
[2] Means ± SD.
[3] Performed on ln values.
Note: **significant differences are shown in bold italics.**

V. Some outcome variables

Table 5.5 describes some outcome variables. The last Hct value was recorded at a median of seven days (hinges: 5-8) from intervention in 94% of operated patients; the median value was 34% (hinges: 31-37%).

The same values were observed in patients transfused with red units. Higher discharge values were observed in hospitals located in central-northern Europe (Figure 5.30).

In transfused patients, the overall fall in Hct was −5.9% ± 11.1 after transfusion of 3.4 ± 2.2 red units (means ± SD). Among hospitals the smallest and largest Hct falls were −0.9% ± 15.1 and −9.8 ± 4.6 after transfusion of 3.7 ± 1.9 and 4.5 ± 2.9 red units, respectively. In untransfused patients, the overall Hct fall was −6.8% ± 13.5, ranging among hospitals from −5.4% ± 13.1 to −10.8% ± 11.3.

159

Table 5.5. CABG: outcome variables

	PA	ED*	IG	DKC	DKA	EC	EA*	GBG	PB	NLA	FC	DB	FB	GBF	ID	BA	BB	BC	DA	GBA	IH
Last Hct																					
% Po with	23	•	96	98	97	93	91	100	98	100	100	100	100	99	100	99	97	98	100	100	89
%, median value	33		31	35	35	32	27	32	38	36	32	34.5	33	32	31	34	33	33	35	34	32
range	28-39		25-40	29-48	30-44	22-44	21-37	28-41	28-46	27-44	26-42	24-43	20-42	25-44	24-42	25-42	26-46	21-42	27-48	25-47	25-43
Complication of allogeneic autologous transfusion (% Pt)					1.7								1.9			1.5					
Reoperation % Po				9.7	1.7	1.7		8.3	2.3	1.6		8.8		1.4		4.0	2.6			8.3	7.3
Mortality % Po						3.4	9.1		11.6		16.7		7.9	1.4		1.3	2.6	3.0		5.6	
LOS median days	8		10	12	9	15	19	13	17	12	12	10	16	9	16	16	13	15	18	9	22
range	7-52		4-22	2-22	7-15	8-46	9-76	6-37	8-57	9-26	4-32	3-20	6-56	6-34	11-53	8-80	3-24	4-33	7-78	7-66	1-60

Po = patient operated.
Pt = patients transfused.
• = not calculated due to the small size of patient sample.
Hospital code and * = less than 20 patients.

Complications of blood transfusion were reported by only three hospitals (Table 5.6).

Table 5.6. CABG: complications of transfusion

Type	Involved patient number	Transfused[1] patient number	Hospitals reporting / all hospitals
Allogeneic transfusion			
haemolytic reaction[2]	1	59	1/20
fever/rigors	2	120	2/20

Type	Involved patient number	Donating patient number[3]	Hospitals reporting / all hospitals
Autologous donation			
anaemia	1	73	1/15
not specified	2	16	1/15

[1] Transfused with blood components.
[2] Due to an anti-Jka antibody.
[3] IBS technique excluded.

Complications of surgery

Reoperated patients had a postoperative blood loss, and a number of red units transfused falling above the upper quartile of the overall patient distribution and had a frequency of subsequent death of 17% (6/35) (Table 5.7). Six of 28 patients (21%) who died previously underwent a reoperation.

Deaths were more than twice as frequent in females as in males. Age, blood loss and number of red units transfused in patients who died fell above the upper quartile of overall patient distribution, whereas preoperative and last Hct values fell in the majority of the cases below the lower quartile of the distribution. Features characterizing reoperated patients were: high blood loss volumes and the number of transfused red units falling above the upper quartile of the distribution.

Median LOS before surgery was three days (hinges: 2-5) and after surgery 10 days (hinges: 7-12). No important differences in preoperative LOS were found between the hospitals of the two broad geographic areas (Figure 5.31); however, four of the five showing a median preoperative LOS of five or more days were located in the Mediterranean area.

VI. Costs

Overall product cost per operated patient was ECU 413 (Figure 5.32). The lowest and highest costs observed among hospitals were ECU 19 and 643 per operated patient, respectively (Figure 5.33). The product dominating cost varied according to the hospital (plasma in DKA, albumin in GBF, for example).

161

Table 5.7. CABG: complications of surgery

	Hospital number	Patient number	Age, years	Gender M:F	Preoperative Hct %	Blood loss, L perioperative	Blood loss, L postoperative	Red units per patient	Last Hct %	Postoperative LOS, days	Death: day number after surgery [1]
Reoperation for bleeding											
recorded in	12/21	35 35/1 166	57 (53-72)	4:1	44 (31-48) 30/35	0.8 (0.5-2.3) 9/35	1.7 (0.4-13.0) (23/35)	7 (1-53)	35 (25-48) 26/35	10 (0-64)	10 (0-64) 6/35
deaths											
recorded in	10/21	28 28/1 166	66 (36-82)	2:1	40 (32-53) 19/21	1.2 (0.2-2.3) 10/28	0.9 (0.3-13.0) 16/28	7 (1-53) 26/28	30 (20-33) 12/28		6 (0-64)

[1] Median (range).

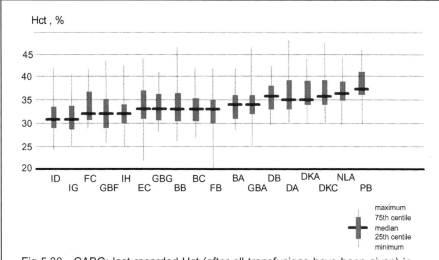

Fig 5.30.- CABG: last recorded Hct (after all transfusions have been given) in patients transfused with red units in each hospital. Each distribution refers to twenty or more patients

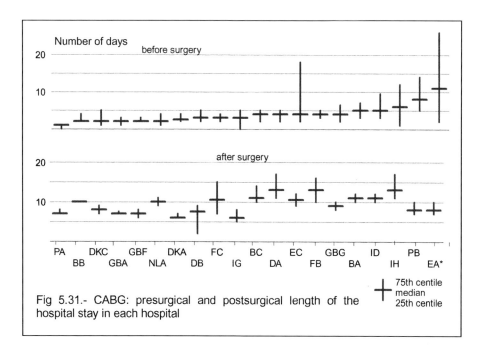

Fig 5.31.- CABG: presurgical and postsurgical length of the hospital stay in each hospital

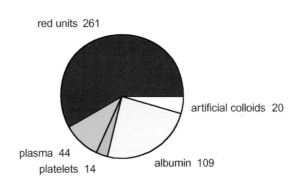

Fig 5.32. - CABG: overall estimated costs according to the product used. Values indicate ECUs per patient operated

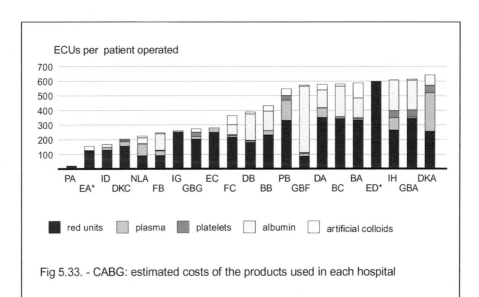

Fig 5.33. - CABG: estimated costs of the products used in each hospital

VII. Summary and comments on CABG

CABG patients received red units (88%), albumin (54%), artificial colloids (48%), plasma (39%) and platelets (8%). However, these proportions of patients differed greatly among hospitals, even within a country: from 17 to 100% for red units, 0 to 100% for albumin, 0 to 100% for artificial colloids, 0 to 100% for plasma and 0 to 38% for platelets. Substantial variations were also observed in the median amount of product administered to recipients: from one to five for red units, 21 to 226 g for albumin, 0.5 to 4 L for artificial colloids, 1 to 10 units for plasma, four to eight units for platelets. In some hospitals (BA, BB, DA), the higher the number of products used, the higher the proportion of recipients and the amount of product administered.

In two thirds of the hospitals the proportion of patients transfused with red units was 90% or higher; however, for CABG the difference between the highest and lowest users of red units (17 and 100%) was among the largest interhospital variations found in this study. In the hospital (PA) where the proportion of transfused patients was lowest, none of the studied variables showed values different from those observed in other hospitals. On the contrary, among hospitals where the great majority of operated patients were transfused, there were some with younger patients (PB, GBF), with patients with higher preoperative Hct values (PB, GBF, GBA) and with a higher proportion of patients undergoing the saphenous vein graft only (PB, BC, GBA). These findings suggest that again the hospital itself is the major source of the variations. However it remains possible, since this study did not seek to collect all data of possible relevance, that other factors (such as a special selection of patients in some hospitals, severity of illness and comorbidity of patients, the number of vessels bypassed and other surgical aspects) may affect blood use and explain some of the variations.

In a third of the hospitals, some variables were found to affect patient transfusion, such as age, preoperative Hct and blood loss. However, patient transfusion differed among hospitals, after adjustment for age and preoperative Hct, and after further adjustment for blood loss (although the latter was feasible only in two hospitals where adequate blood loss data were available). Recorded blood loss in CABG appeared to affect transfusion to a smaller extent than in other surgical procedures. This may be due in part to under-recording of losses, or to transfusion without reference to estimated blood loss. Saphenous vein graft appeared to be associated with a higher patient transfusion than mammary or mammary artery plus saphenous grafts. Any influence of different graft procedures may well be confounded by other factors, including the identified 'hospital effect'.

Preoperative Hct value and blood loss did not affect the units transfused in hospitals using little or no autotransfusion, whereas it did in hospitals with moderate or high autotransfusion use, since the availability of IBS allowed retrieval of shed blood. Hospitals differed also in the number of units per patient transfused, even after adjustment for age, preoperative Hct and blood loss.

Also, the use of autotransfusion varied among hospitals: the proportion of operated patients transfused with autologous red units ranged from 0 to 100%. The proportion of patients transfused with autologous units in hospitals of central-northern Europe was half that observed in hospitals of the Mediterranean area.

The threshold for postoperative transfusion was a mean Hct of 28% ±2.9.

Plasma transfusion, as in a previous study, [2] occurred in nearly all hospitals, although in different proportions of operated patients. In six of 21 hospitals, 50% or more of operated patients were transfused with plasma, whereas 10% or less in only three hospitals. Furthermore, one quarter of the patients received one or two units of plasma, a dose deemed ineffective in the treatment of coagulation disorders. [12] Information available did not allow adequate evaluation of the appropriateness of plasma transfusion; however its frequent use does not seem consistent with the presence of factors that constitute accepted indications for the transfusion of plasma. Liquid plasma may have been transfused for volume replacement, as explicitly indicated by the reasons, although few, documented in the clinical record. Furthermore, three quarters of plasma recipients were transfused with red cell concentrates during the same 24-hour period, strongly suggesting that 'reconstituted' whole blood from the two components was being employed. The proportion of patients transfused with plasma was twice as great in hospitals of central-northern Europe as in the Mediterranean countries.

More than one quarter of patients received platelet concentrates in three hospitals. The use of platelets and cryoprecipitates was mainly observed in hospitals in central-northern Europe.

Interhospital differences in the use of colloids may in part be explained by the limited availability of these products in some countries: the proportion of albumin recipients was twice as high in the hospitals of central-northern Europe as in those of the Mediterranean area, and the use of artificial colloids five times higher. Furthermore, diversities from hospital to hospital were observed in both the proportion of recipients and amount of colloids given even within a country where the health care organization and product availability would be expected to be homogeneous.

6.0. Abdominal aorta aneurysmectomy (AAA)

Abdominal aorta aneurysm is one of the most common and dangerous arterial aneurysms. Its resection is accompanied by an appreciable extension of life. More than 95% of abdominal aorta aneurysms are due to atherosclerosis and occur mainly in the sixth to seventh decade of age. Frequency in males outnumbers that in females by 6:1. Mortality rate is usually <0.5% and is primarily due to associated lesions of atherosclerosis that complicate postsurgical recovery.

Case report forms were available from 693 patients in 23 hospitals and 10 countries: 456 (66%) in 14 hospitals in six central-northern European countries and 237 (34%) in nine hospitals in four Mediterranean countries (Figure 6.1).

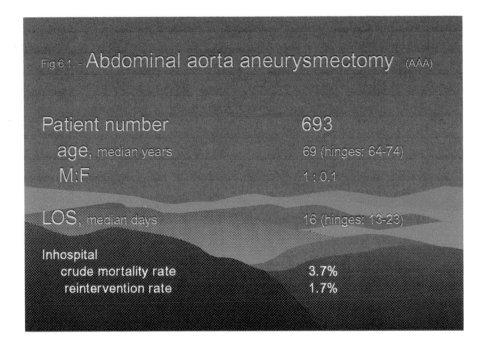

Fig 6.1. - Abdominal aorta aneurysmectomy (AAA)

Patient number	693
age, median years	69 (hinges: 64-74)
M:F	1 : 0.1
LOS, median days	16 (hinges: 13-23)
Inhospital	
crude mortality rate	3.7%
reintervention rate	1.7%

I. Patient data and some variables related to surgery

Table 6.1 reports, by hospital, the number, age and gender of patients, and the values of some variables related to surgery. The median age was between 68 and 70 years in more than three quarters of the hospitals. The M:F ratio was high and in some hospitals only males were reported.

The median preoperative Hct value was 42% (hinges: 38-45%), being 42% or higher in the majority of hospitals.

Of operated patients, 73% received a drug acting on the coagulation system. 72% of patients received an anticoagulant or an anti-platelet drug and 1% also a haemostatic drug. Figures 6.2 and 6.3 depict, globally and by hospital, the percentage of operated patients receiving a drug according to the time in relation to surgery.

167

Table 6.1. AAA: patient data and some variables related to surgery

	DKA	IG	GRE	EC*	EA*	GBF*	PB*	IA	GBA	FC	FB	BB	IH*	ID	NLB	BA	DB*	GBE*	ED*	BC	DKC	DA	NLA
Patient number	41	41	50	13	3	1	1	58	55	32	49	61	13	49	21	48	8	8	9	27	57	26	22
Age, median years	68	70	70	70				70	68	70	69	69	67	66	69	67	67	67	70	69	71	68	68
range	52-88	56-81	55-91	55-81				51-88	50-82	46-82	47-87	56-87	55-77	51-84	51-84	46-81	44-82	60-77	63-81	51-86	45-83	47-83	50-82
M:F ratio	4.1	19	49	12				5.4	3.2	15.0	7.2	29.5	all M	15.4	4.2	all M	7.0	3.0	all M	all M	3.7	all M	21
Preoperative Hct																							
% Po with	88	95	86	61				96	89	100	100	100	100	92	100	98	62	100	89	96	93	77	100
%, median value	42	42	43	39				40	42	42	42	40	44	40	43	43	47	45	42	39	40	38	43
range	29-49	31-47	32-50	33-48				29-47	33-52	33-50	32-52	24-50	27-49	29-48	38-50	27-52	37-50	36-52	38-47	24-51	32-48	31-48	37-49
Drugs[1]																							
% Po	78	100	2	100				3	100	34	96	98	100	31	100	100	100	100	44	67	100	100	100
Anaesthesia																							
Regional or combined % Po	54	4.9							96	3.1					81	67		37			95		73
Graft																							
% Po: aorto-bifemoral	34.1	4.9	36	53.8	•	•	•	19.0	34.5	31.2	12.2	19.7	30.8	26.5	47.6	29.2	12.5	25	22.2	55.5	17.5	30.8	45.4
aorto-bi-iliac	24.4	65.8	10	15.4	•			32.7	20.0	34.4	32.6	55.7		65.3	4.8	66.7	87.5	75	22.2	44.5	7.0	46.1	18.2
aorto-aortic T-T	41.5	29.3	54	30.8				48.3	45.5	34.4	55.2	24.6	69.2	8.2	47.6	4.1			55.6		75.5	23.1	36.4
Duration of surgery																							
% Po with	73	41	76	100	•	•	•	48	87		100	82	100		86	73		62	100	82	98		77
median minutes	180	180	240	210				135	200		210	160	180		150	210		160	300	320	145		210
range	85-335	180-180	150-360	170-310				60-300	65-380		90-330	90-315	120-240		90-250	105-360		85-195	150-380	210-480	65-250		135-255
Blood loss																							
perioperative																							
% Po with	68	85	100	92	•	•	•		96	41	33	82		100	100	4	100	75	100	93	98	100	100
median L	2.0	0.8	1.6	1.2	•	•	•		1.0	1.2	1.3	0.5		1.1	1.1	•	2.0	1.9	1.6	2.2	1.5	1.5	1.5
range	0.4-5.0	0.3-3.0	0.3-5.5	0.8-3.2					0.2-3.0	0.1-3.0	0.3-3.0	0.0-2.5		0.2-3.2	0.2-3.2	•	0.4-4.0	1.0-14.9	0.5-12.9	0.6-15.0	0.3-4.5	0.4-4.5	0.6-3.0
postoperative																							
% Po with	46	46	2	61				20	7	62	55	97	92	24	24	6				11		23	50
median L	0.2	0.2	•	•				0.1	•	0.3	0.2	0.3	0.4	•	•	•				•		1.1	0.0
range	0.1-0.8	0.1-0.8						0.0-0.8		0.0-3.5	0.0-1.8	0.0-6.0	0.12-2.0									0.2-4.0	0.0-0.3

[1] Only anticoagulants were administered.

Po = patients operated.

• = quantities not calculated due to the small sample size.

* = hospital with less than 20 patients.

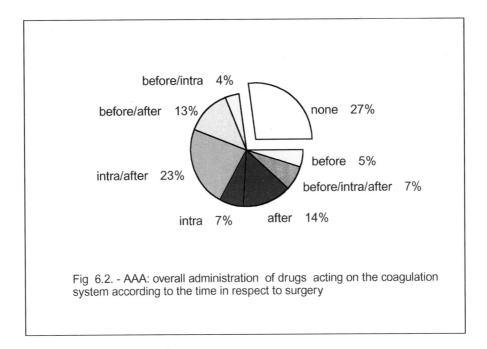

Fig 6.2. - AAA: overall administration of drugs acting on the coagulation system according to the time in respect to surgery

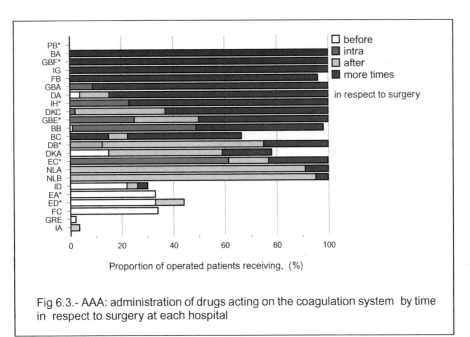

Proportion of operated patients receiving, (%)

Fig 6.3.- AAA: administration of drugs acting on the coagulation system by time in respect to surgery at each hospital

Figure 6.4 shows the overall percentage of recipients according to type of drug.

Anaesthesia was general in 71%, combined in 27% and regional in 2% of the cases. In some hospitals (NLA, NLB, DKA, DKC, GBA, BA), regional or combined anaesthesia was used in the majority of patients.

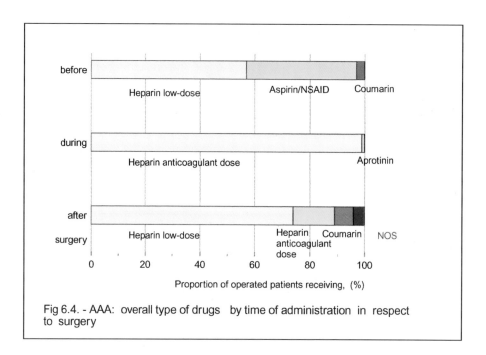

Fig 6.4. - AAA: overall type of drugs by time of administration in respect to surgery

39% of operated patients underwent aorto-aortic graft, 35% aorto-bi-iliac, and 26% aorto-bifemoral graft.

Information on duration of surgery was available in 65% of patients and for the majority of them in three quarters of hospitals. The median time was 180 minutes (hinges: 150-240). Extremes between hospitals were 135 and 320 minutes.

Perioperative blood loss was recorded in 63% patients and postoperative loss in 27%. The median volume was 1.3 L (hinges: 0.8-2.0) perioperatively (Figure 6.5.) and 0.25 L (hinges: 0.12-0.46) postoperatively.

II. Transfusion data

Table 6.2 shows that 16 of 23 hospitals used all three products, six used blood components and artificial colloids, and one (DKA) used blood components and albumin. In the latter hospital, blood components and albumin were used in all the surgical procedures. In five (NL, D, B, F, E)

out of nine countries, all of the hospitals used the same combination of products. Table 6.2 also shows, by hospital, the percentage of recipients by product and the quantities of product per recipient.

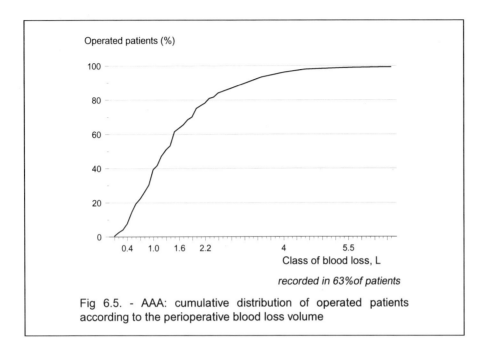

Fig 6.5. - AAA: cumulative distribution of operated patients according to the perioperative blood loss volume

II.1.0. *Red units*

82% of patients were transfused with 2 663 red units. Among hospitals, the proportion of transfused patients varied from 64 to 100%. The proportion of patients transfused in central-northern European countries was similar to that observed in the Mediterranean area.

In recipients, the median number of red units was three (hinges: 2-6) and varied among hospitals from two to seven. The cumulative distribution of the number of red units in operated patients is reported in Figure 6.6. Of operated patients, 29% received a number of red units higher than four.

II.1.1. *Allogeneic and autologous transfusion*

In all 372 patients were transfused with 1 673 allogeneic red units, 90 with 205 autologous units, and 111 with 315 autologous and 470 allogeneic red units (Figure 6.7, and Table 0.3, Part I). Wide interhospital differences were evident in the use of autologous as well as allogeneic red units (Figure 6.8). In hospitals of central-northern Europe, the proportion of patients transfused with autologous units was less than half that in the Mediterranean area (RR = 0.4 (0.3 to 0.5)).

IBS, alone or associated with other techniques, was the method most widely used (Figure 6.9). Nearly four times more red units were provided by IBS than by other autotransfusion techniques (Figure 6.7).

Table 6.2. AAA: transfusion data

	DKA	IG	GRE	EC*	EA*	GBF*	PB*	IA	GBA	FC	FB	BB	IH*	ID	NLB	BA	DB*	GBE*	ED*	BC	DKC	DA	NLA
Red units — patients																							
transfused/operated (%)	97.6	82.9	100	100	100	100	100	63.8	65.4	68.7	73.5	75.4	69.2	79.6	76.2	83.3	87.5	87.5	88.9	96.3	98.2	100	90.9
units per transfused patient — median	4	2	6	•	•	•	•	2	2	3.5	3	2.5	•	3	4	3	•	•	•	6	4	7	3
hinges	3-6	2-5	4-9					1-3	2-3	3-11	2-4	2-4		2-5	2-4	2-5				4-9	3-5.5	4-12	2-4
Plasma — patients																							
transfused/operated (%)	12.2	21.9	42	46.1	33.3		100	10.3	3.6	12.5	8.2	31.1	38.5	24.5	28.6	4.2	50	12.5	55.5	77.8	14	65.4	100
units per transfused patient — median	4	1	3	•	•		•	2	•	4.5	•	3	•	3	3	•	•	•	•	8	4	3	6
hinges	3-4	1-3	2-6					2-4		3.5-5.5		1-4		2-6	2-4					6-10	4-5	2-5	4-8
Platelets — patients																							
transfused/operated (%)	4.9			7.7					3.6	3.1	2				9.5			12.5		11.1	7	3.8	
units per transfused patient — median	•			•					•	•	•				•					10			
hinges										•	•									8-12			
Cryoprecipitate — patients																							
transfused/operated (%)				7.7					1.8	3.1		1.6			4.8			12.5		7.4			
Albumin — patients																							
administered/operated (%)	75.6			76.9	100	100	100	27.6	47.3	34.4	85.7	100	15.4	2	61.9	58.3	50	25	11.1	100	42.1	69.2	59
grams per recipient — median	72							31.5	41	52	41.5	122	•	•	61	42	•	•	•	122	26	77.5	41
hinges	26-134							11-43	21-62	41-61	41-82	88-199			41-61	21-82				83-183	13-38	51-182	21-41
Colloids — patients																							
administered/operated (%)		41.5	16	76.9	100	100	100	39.6	78.2	96.9	73.5	50.8	53.8	26.5	95.2	100	100	87.5	77.8	96.3	98.2	100	90.9
L per recipient — median		0.5	1					0.5	1	1.5	1	0.5	•	1	1.2	1	•	•	•	1.9	0.5	1.5	0.5
hinges		0.1-0.5	0.5-1.2					0.5-0.5	0.7-1.5	1.0-2.0	0.5-1.0	0.5-0.5		1.0-1.0	1.0-1.7	0.5-3.0				1.0-3.0	0.5-1.0	0.5-2.0	0.5-1.0
Patients for whom the number of autologous blood units was partly or completely not reported (% operated)											2.0	3.3						12.5					

Hospitals are aggregated according to products used.

• = quantities not calculated due to the small patient sample.

Hospital code and * = less than 20 patients.

[1] Autotransfusion use.

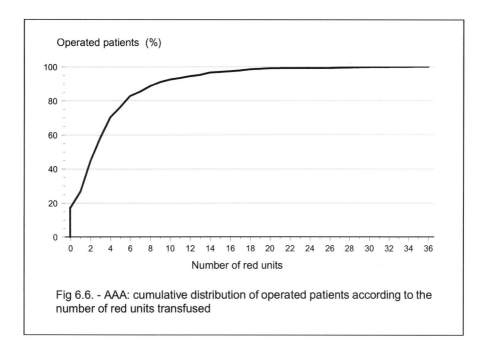

Fig 6.6. - AAA: cumulative distribution of operated patients according to the number of red units transfused

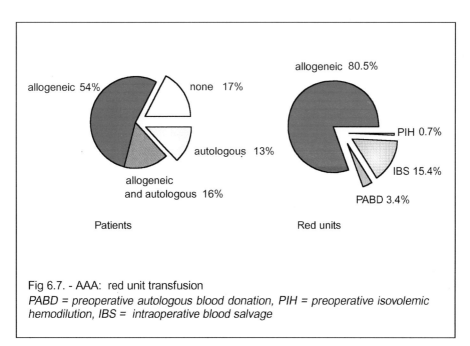

Fig 6.7. - AAA: red unit transfusion
PABD = preoperative autologous blood donation, PIH = preoperative isovolemic hemodilution, IBS = intraoperative blood salvage

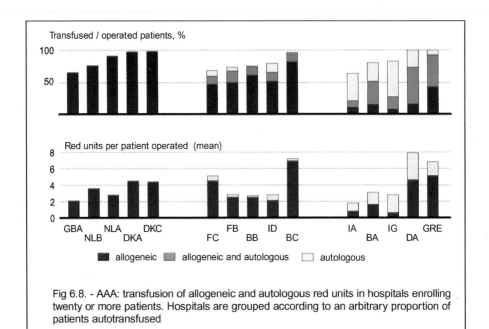

Fig 6.8. - AAA: transfusion of allogeneic and autologous red units in hospitals enrolling twenty or more patients. Hospitals are grouped according to an arbitrary proportion of patients autotransfused

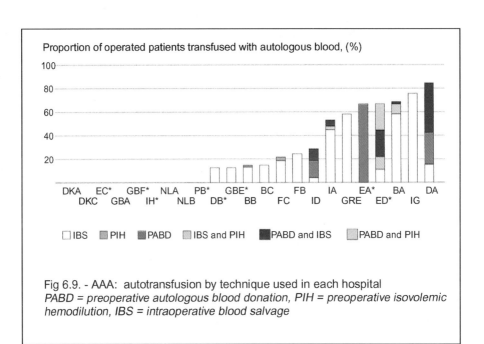

Fig 6.9. - AAA: autotransfusion by technique used in each hospital
PABD = preoperative autologous blood donation, PIH = preoperative isovolemic hemodilution, IBS = intraoperative blood salvage

II.1.2. *Allogeneic whole blood use*

Of transfused red units, 10% were represented by whole blood. In three hospitals (GBF, GBE, and BA), they accounted for more than 50% of red units transfused (Figure 6.10).

A comparison between the use of red units of Sanguis hospitals and that of two other studies is shown in Figure 6.11.

II.1.3. *Time of transfusion*

Transfusion episodes (Figure 6.12) were not infrequent after surgery, although involving a small proportion of patients. In some hospitals (NLB, ID, DB, FC), up to one quarter of patients were transfused in the postoperative period (Figure 6.13).

The mean number of transfusion episodes was 1.3 per patient transfused.

II.2.0. *Platelets*

In all 117 platelet concentrates were transfused to 18 patients (3%) in 10 of 23 hospitals. The majority of hospitals using platelets was in central-northern European countries. The median number was five (hinges: 4-8). 26% of the units were from apheresis, nearly all of them in one hospital (BC).

In nearly all hospitals using platelet concentrates, cryoprecipitates were also used (Table 6.2).

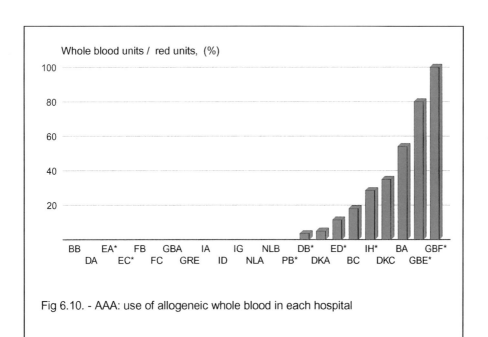

Fig 6.10. - AAA: use of allogeneic whole blood in each hospital

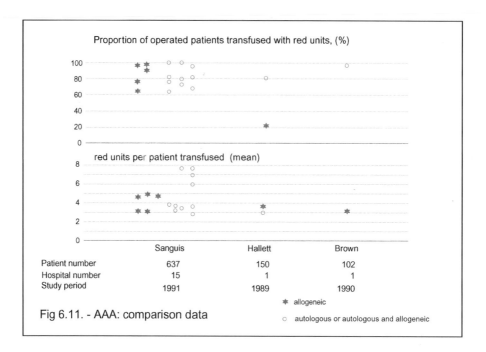

Fig 6.11. - AAA: comparison data

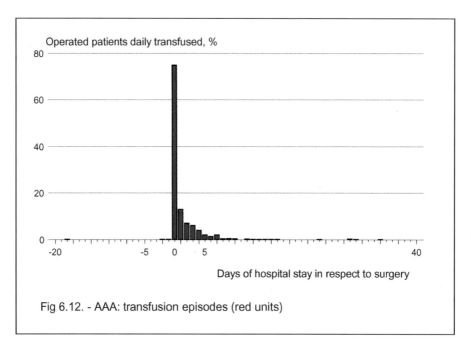

Fig 6.12. - AAA: transfusion episodes (red units)

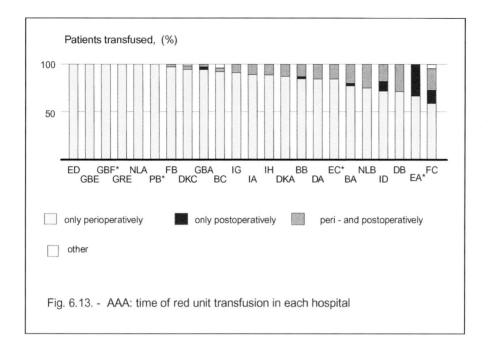

Fig. 6.13. - AAA: time of red unit transfusion in each hospital

II.3.0. *Plasma*

In all 824 plasma units were transfused to 181 (26%) patients in all hospitals except in GBF (Figure 6.14). The percentage of plasma recipients, varying among hospitals from 0 to 100, did not differ between the two broad geographic areas.

In recipients, the median number of units was four (hinges: 2-5) and varied among hospitals from one to eight. Of plasma units transfused, 3% were autologous (ED, and DA which accounted for 2.7%), 55% were fresh frozen, 15% apheresis (BC accounting for 13%) and 27% liquid (DKA, EC, GRE, NLB, PB, and NLA alone accounting for 17%).

Of 176 recipients of allogeneic plasma, 158 also received red cell concentrates, 85% of them within the same 24-hour period.

II.4.0. *Cryoprecipitates*

In all 37 units were given to eight patients in seven hospitals, six of them in central-northern Europe. The median number of units was three (hinges: 2-7)

II.5.0. *Albumin*

In all 30 444 g of albumin were administered to 320 patients (46%) in 17 of 23 hospitals, 13 of them in central-northern Europe (Figure 6.15). 41% of the recipients and 58% of the amount used were from three hospitals (BB, BC, FB). As a consequence, the proportion of recipients in

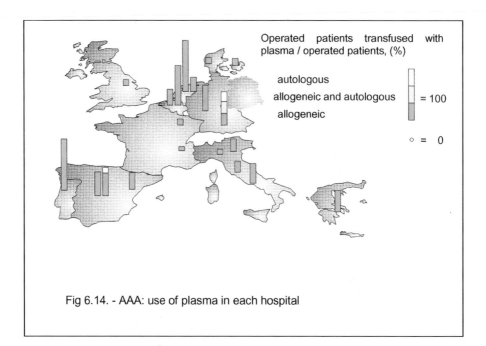

Fig 6.14. - AAA: use of plasma in each hospital

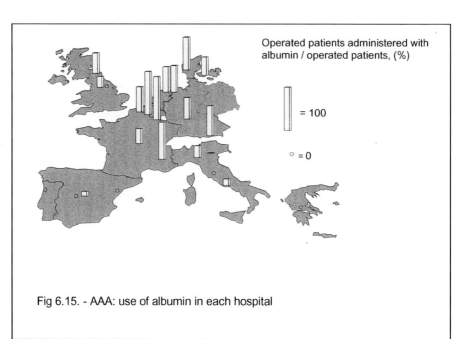

Fig 6.15. - AAA: use of albumin in each hospital

central-northern Europe was 10 times higher than in the Mediterranean area (RR = 10 (7 to 13)). In recipients, the median amount was 61 g (hinges: 28-122). Hospitals using albumin differed widely in both the percentage of recipients (range 2 to 100%), and in the amount given to recipients (range of the medians: 26 to 122 g).

II.6.0. *Artificial colloids*

In all 673 L of artificial colloids were administered to 442 patients (64%) in almost all hospitals (Figure 6.16). In recipients, the median volume was 1.0 L (hinges: 0.5-1.5). A high use of artificial colloids was observed in four hospitals (BA, BC, DA, FC) which reported 39% of the recipients and 56% of the volume used. As a consequence, the proportion of recipients in hospitals of central-northern Europe was three times higher than that observed in the Mediterranean area (RR = 3 (2 to 3)).

11% of artificial colloids were given as HES, 19% as dextrans and 70% as gelatin. Variability among hospitals in the type and amount of colloid per operated patient is shown in Figure 6.17.

In recipients, the median volume given was 0.5 L (hinges: 0.5-1.0) for both HES and dextrans, and 1.0 L (hinges: 0.5-2.0) for gelatin. The median volumes of the latter colloid varied among hospitals from 0.5 to 3.0 L.

The variety of products used by the hospitals is shown in Figure 6.18 and that in hospitals aggregated according to country in Figure 6.19.

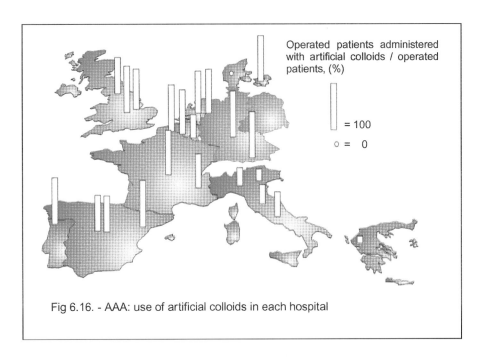

Fig 6.16. - AAA: use of artificial colloids in each hospital

179

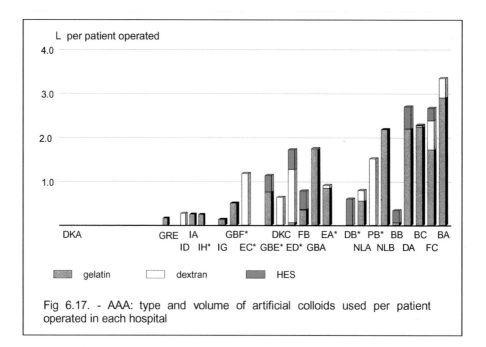

Fig 6.17. - AAA: type and volume of artificial colloids used per patient operated in each hospital

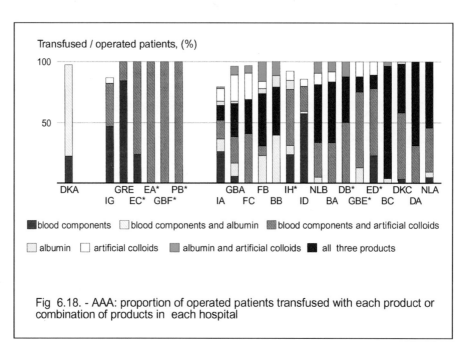

Fig 6.18. - AAA: proportion of operated patients transfused with each product or combination of products in each hospital

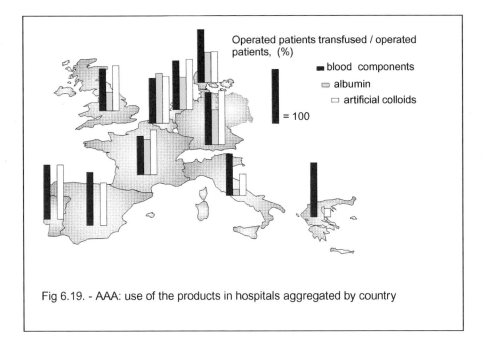

Fig 6.19. - AAA: use of the products in hospitals aggregated by country

III. Reasons for transfusion documented in the medical record

III.1. *Red units*

A reason was documented in 29% of recipients and in 17 of 23 hospitals (Figure 6.20). Reasons were presence of bleeding (19%), a low Hct value (7%), volume replacement (2%) and a low Hct value with presence of bleeding (1%).

III.2. *Plasma*

Reasons were given in 37% of patients from 10 hospitals. Bleeding and volume replacement were reported for 17% of the recipients. A PT value was also found in a total of 17% of patients, two thirds of them in Belgian hospitals.

III.3. *Platelets*

A reason for transfusion (mainly bleeding) was given in 25% of the recipients.

III.4. *Albumin*

Reasons were given in 22% of the recipients and in 11 hospitals. In the majority of the cases, they were volume replacement and/or bleeding.

III.5. *Artificial colloids*

Reasons were given in 17% of recipients from 11 hospitals, in the majority for volume replacement.

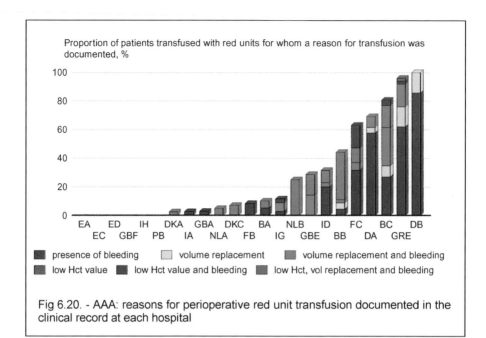

Fig 6.20. - AAA: reasons for perioperative red unit transfusion documented in the clinical record at each hospital

IV. Variables associated with red unit transfusion

IV.1. *Transfused versus untransfused patients*

A higher age, a lower presurgical Hct value and a higher blood loss volume characterized the sub-set of patients transfused (Table 6.3). 42% of untransfused patients were from a few hospitals (IA, FC, GBA).

IV.2. *Preoperatively transfused patients*

Three patients were preoperatively transfused. They were two males and one female, aged 65, 69 and 74 years. Pretransfusion Hct was 21, 24, and 30%; after transfusion of three and five units, post-transfusion Hct was 36 and 44% (values available in two patients). Two patients died, 7 and 11 days after surgery.

IV.3. *Perioperatively transfused patients*

Indicator: proportion of perioperatively transfused patients (mean percentage $\pm$ SE)

Hospitals: eight (53%) of 15 with 20 or more patients

Patients: 344 (56%) of 611, after exclusion of females (due to the small sample size), reinterventions and deaths

Factors: age, preintervention Hct, graft, blood loss

The effect of a factor on the probability of a patient being transfused cannot be estimated when all or nearly all patients (90% or more) are transfused. For this reason only about half of the

Table 6.3. AAA: comparison between patients transfused with red units and not transfused during the hospital stay

	Patients transfused			Patients not transfused	95% confidence interval of the difference[2]
	allogeneic	allogeneic and autologous	autologous		
Patient number	372	111	89	121	
Age, years[1]	*70 (65-75)*	69 (63-73)	67 (62-71)	*66 (60-71)*	*−2 to −6*
M:F	7.1	17.5	28.7	8.3	0.3 to 2
Hct preintervention,[1] %	*41 (38-44)*	40 (37-43)	43 (39-45)	*43 (40-45)*	*1.1 to 2.9*
Percentage of patients with	90	95	96	99	
Anaesthesia, regional and/or combined, % Po	39	13.5	10	25	
Anticoagulants, % Po	80	62.2	61	69	
Haemostatic, % Po		1.8	1.1		
Duration of surgery, minutes	180 (145-240)	225 (180-270)	180 (170-220)	180 (130-205)	
Percentage of patients with	73	58	52	59	
Blood loss,[1] L perioperative	*1.4 (0.9-2.0)*	1.8 (1.6-2.0)	0.9 (0.7-2.3)	*0.6 (0.4-1.0)*	*0.37 to 0.56*[3]
Percentage of patients with	62	15	16	40	
Percentage of patients transfused with					
plasma	33.1	37.8	11.2		
albumin	54.6	45.0	21.3	40.0	
artificial colloids	66.4	61.3	53.9	65.0	
PABD, % patients		97.3	100		
Stated reason for transfusion, % Pt	26	53	9.2		
Reintervention for bleeding, % Po	2.69	1.8			
In-hospital crude mortality rate, % Po	5.65	3.6		0.83	
Last Hct,[1] %	34 (32-37)	34 (30-37)	35 (31-38)	34 (32-37)	
Percentage of patients with	95	85	98	98	
Hospital stay,[1] day number	16 (12-21)	23 (16-29)	19 (14-22)	15 (12-21)	
before surgery	4 (2-7)	6 (2-11)	7 (4-12)	4 (2-8)	
after surgery	11 (8-14)	13 (10-19)	10 (9-12)	10 (9-12)	

Po = patients operated.
Pt = patients transfused.
[1] Median (hinges).
[2] Between patients not transfused and transfused with allogeneic red units, after exclusion of deaths and reinterventions.
[3] Performed on ln values.
Note: **significant differences are shown in bold italics.**

hospitals (and patients) could be studied. A comparison between patients of hospitals excluded from analysis and those included showed no difference in patient age, but a higher proportion (+10%) of patients with a preoperative Hct value <40% and a higher proportion (+23%) of patients with blood loss volumes higher than 1.7 L.

The probability of a patient being transfused (Part I, Figure 0.14) increased with increasing age (difference between the highest and lowest age class = +18%), with increasing blood loss volumes (difference between the highest and lowest class = +23%), and decreased with increasing preoperative Hct values (difference between the highest and lowest class = −27%). The type of graft did not seem to affect the probability of a patient of being transfused (aorto-aortic graft 70%±3.2, bifemoral 70%±1.5, bi-iliac 76%±1.0).

In hospitals with a high use of autotransfusion, the probability of transfusion did not decrease with increasing preoperative Hct values, suggesting that when autotransfusion is often used, this variable was no longer predictive. This is confirmed also by the much higher probability of patient transfusion even at preoperative Hct values higher than 43% in comparison with that observed in hospitals using autotransfusion less regularly (74%±1.9 versus 56%±1.5).

Age affected the probability of patients being transfused in seven of eight hospitals, preoperative Hct value in six of eight hospitals (but in one case the trend was opposite) (Figure 6.21), and blood loss in two of three hospitals (Figure 6.22).

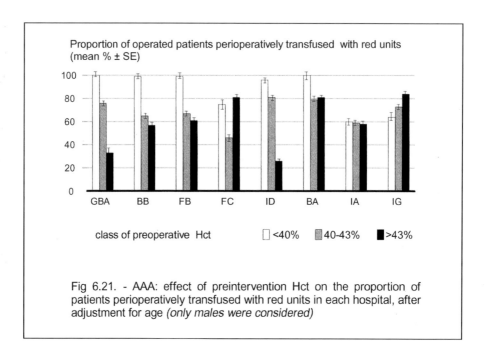

Fig 6.21. - AAA: effect of preintervention Hct on the proportion of patients perioperatively transfused with red units in each hospital, after adjustment for age *(only males were considered)*

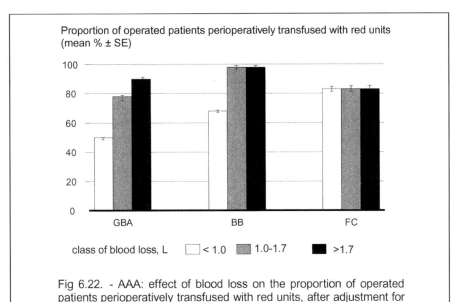

Fig 6.22. - AAA: effect of blood loss on the proportion of operated patients perioperatively transfused with red units, after adjustment for age *(only males are considered)*

The bi-iliac graft was associated with a higher probability of transfusion in three of eight hospitals, and lower probability in one hospital; the bifemoral graft with a higher patient transfusion in 1 hospital, the aorto-aortic in one hospital, and both the aorto-aortic and bifemoral graft in one hospital (Figure 6.23).

After adjustment for the effect of age and preoperative Hct, hospitals still differed in patient transfusion (Figure 6.24), ranging from $60\% \pm 1.6$ to $88\% \pm 1.6$. No adjustment for blood loss was feasible due to the small number of available data.

In ascending order, the differences in the proportion of patients transfused attributable to age were 18%, to blood loss 23% and to preoperative Hct 27%.

A summary of the variables implied in patient transfusion within hospitals is given in Figure 6.23.

IV.4. *Perioperative transfusion of red units*

Indicator: red units per patient perioperatively transfused (mean number $\pm$ SE)

Hospitals: 13 (87%) of 15 with 20 or more patients

Patients: 419 (68%) of 611, after exclusion of females (due to the small sample size), reinterventions and deaths

Factors: age, preintervention Hct, graft, blood loss

On average, the mean number of red units per patient transfused increased with increasing blood loss volumes (difference between the highest and lowest class of blood loss + 3.5 units),

185

	age, years	graft			presurgical Hct, %	blood loss, L
	>65 vs <65	AA	Bifem	Bisil	>43 vs <40	>1.0 vs 1.7
BA	⇧	⇧	⇧		⇩	/
BB	⇧		⇧		⇩	⇧
FB	⇧			⇧	⇩	/
FC	⇧			⇩		
GBA	⇧	⇧			⇩	⇧
IA	⇧			⇧		/
IG	⇧				⬆	?
ID				⇧	⇩	/

⇧ increase   ⇩ decrease   blank = no variation

/ = data not available   ? = poor sample size

Fig 6.23. - AAA: effect of some variables on the proportion of patients perioperatively transfused with red units in each hospital, after adjustment for age *(only males were considered)* AA = aorto-aortic, Bifem = bi-femoral, Bisil = bis-iliac graft

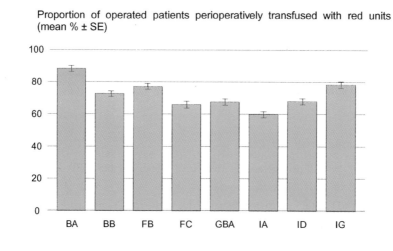

Proportion of operated patients perioperatively transfused with red units (mean % ± SE)

Fig 6.24. - AAA: probability of a patient being perioperatively transfused with red units in each hospital, after adjustment for age and preoperative Hct *(only males were considered)*

and decreased with increasing preoperative Hct values (difference between the highest and lowest class of Hct = − 1.6 units). The bifemoral graft was associated with a higher number of units transfused (3.7 ± 0.09 versus 2.6 ± 0.12 (aorto-aortic) or 2.7 ± 0.08 (bi-iliac)).

The number of units transfused in hospitals with high autotransfusion was higher than in hospitals with no autotransfusion only when blood loss was higher than 1 L (4.3 ± 0.09 versus 2.9 ± 0.07).

Age affected the number of units transfused in three of 13 hospitals (not shown), preoperative Hct value in 11 of 13 hospitals (in two cases being opposite to the expected) (Figure 6.25).

The type of graft was the dominant variable in eight of 11 hospitals (although incoherently) (not shown), while blood loss affected the number of units transfused per patient in eight of eight hospitals (Figure 6.26).

Hospitals differed in the number of units transfused, after adjustment for age and preoperative Hct, ranging from 0.7 ± 0.1 to 5.4 ± 0.3 (Figure 6.27), and even further adjustment for blood loss, ranging from 2.1 ± 0.33 to 4.4 ± 0.30 (difference = 2.3 units) (Figure 6.28).

In ascending order, differences in the number of units transfused attributable to preoperative Hct were 1.6 units, to other, unexplored variables 2.3 units, and due to blood loss 3.5 units.

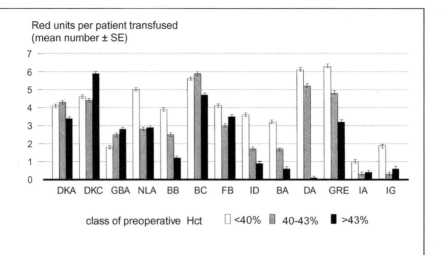

Fig 6.25. - AAA: effect of preoperative Hct on the number of red units perioperatively transfused in each hospital, after adjustment for age *(only males were considered)*

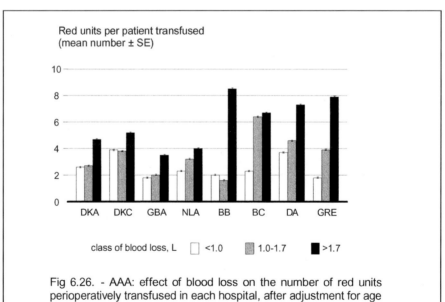

Fig 6.26. - AAA: effect of blood loss on the number of red units perioperatively transfused in each hospital, after adjustment for age *(only males were considered)*

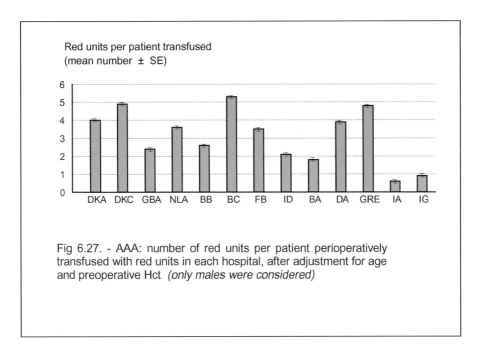

Fig 6.27. - AAA: number of red units per patient perioperatively transfused with red units in each hospital, after adjustment for age and preoperative Hct *(only males were considered)*

IV.5. *Postoperative transfusion*

Profiles of transfused and not transfused patients are shown in Table 6.4, after exclusion of deaths and reinterventions. The threshold for transfusion was an Hct value of $27\% \pm 2.5$ to reach a post-transfusion value of $32\% \pm 3.3$. Two thirds of patients postoperatively transfused were from a few hospitals (ID, BA, BB, FC).

Table 6.4. AAA: some characteristics of patients transfused and not transfused with red units in the postoperative period,[1] after exclusion of deaths and reinterventions

	Patients transfused	Patients not transfused	95% confidence interval of the difference
Patient number	52	556	
Age, years [2]	**70 ± 7.0**	**68 ± 7.8**	**− 4.8 to − 0.4**
Percentage of males	94	90	− 10 to 0.0
Hct pretransfusion, % [2]	27 ± 2.5		
Percentage of patients with	86		
Postoperative blood loss, mL [2]	5.4 ± 1.8	5.3 ± 1.0	0.5 to 1.6 [3]
Percentage of patients with	35	25	
Units per patient transfused [2]	2.9 ± 2		
Last Hct, % [2]	32 ± 3.3	35 ± 4.2	4.3 to − 1.1
Percentage of patients with	50	60	
Postsurgical LOS, days [2]	14.7 ± 6.5	12.1 ± 5.7	

[1] Means ± SD.
[2] From the fourth day after surgery to discharge.
[3] Performed on ln values.

Note: ***significant differences are shown in bold italics.***

V. Outcome variables

Table 6.5 describes some outcome variables. The last Hct value was recorded at a median of six days (hinges: 4-9) after surgery in 94% of operated patients; the median value was 34% (hinges: 31-37%). In nine hospitals, the median value of the last Hct was 33 to 34%, in two hospitals 32% and in the remainder 35 to 38%.

In patients transfused with red units, the median value and hinges of the last Hct were the same as in all operated patients. The last Hct value was recorded after all transfusions had been given at a median of six days (hinges: 3-10) after surgery. Five of the six hospitals where 50% or more of transfused patients had a last Hct value of 35% or higher were located in central-northern European countries (Figure 6.29)

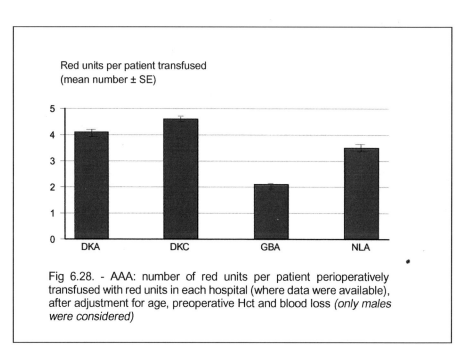

Fig 6.28. - AAA: number of red units per patient perioperatively transfused with red units in each hospital (where data were available), after adjustment for age, preoperative Hct and blood loss *(only males were considered)*

In transfused patients, the overall Hct fall was $-3.0\% \pm 12.8$ with 3.7 ± 2.7 red units transfused (means $\pm$ SD). Among hospitals, the lowest and highest falls were $0\% \pm 12$ and $-9.1\% \pm 5.6$, where 4.1 ± 2.0 and 3.0 ± 1.2 red units were transfused per patient (means $\pm$ SD). In not transfused patients, the overall Hct fall was $-8.3\% \pm 5.9$, the lowest and highest Hct falls being $-5.2\% \pm 3.5$ and $-12.6\% \pm 2.7$.

Table 6.5. AAA: outcome variables

	DKA	IG	GRE	EC*	EA*	GBF*	PB*	IA	GBA	FC	FB	BB	IH*	ID	NLB	BA	DB*	GBE*	ED*	BC	DKC	DA	NLA
Last Hct																							
% Po with	95	98	42	92	*	*	*	98	98	97	100	100	100	100	100	98	100	87	100	96	100	100	91
%, median value	33	34	38	33				34	34	36	33	32	38	33	35	35	34	34	35	34	36	32	36
range	23-41	25-44	30-45	28-39				25-45	26-46	24-42	23-42	17-39	23-48	27-42	29-42	28-42	12-42	28-44	27-41	29-44	27-45	26-42	32-42
Complications of																							
allogeneic												2.1				3.8				3.8			
autologous transfusion (% Pt)																3.0							
Reoperation rate % Po	7.3							1.7		3.1		3.3			9.5			12.5				7.7	
Mortality rate % Po	2.4		4	7.7				6.9		15.6	4.1	3.3			4.7	2.1	25	12.5		14.8			
LOS days, median number	10	20	23	16				15	14	18	14	17	20	29	18	18	13	14	18	16	13	25	13
range	0-20	6-38	3-41	10-31				7-51	8-57	10-45	5-28	4-53	12-40	11-58	11-27	11-51	1-28	1-22	11-27	9-36	6-23	8-49	9-42

• = not calculated due to the small sample size.
Po = patient operated.
Pt = patients transfused.
Hospital code and * = less than 20 patients.

191

Complications of allogeneic and autologous blood transfusion were reported only in Belgian hospitals (Table 6.6).

Table 6.6. AAA: complications of transfusion

	Type	Involved patient number	Transfused[1] patient number	Hospitals reporting	Hospitals reporting / all hospitals
Allogeneic					
	haemolytic reaction[2]	1	47	BB	1/23
	fever/rigors	2		BA, BC	2/23
Autologous					
	allogeneic units were given while autologous ones were available	1	33	BA	1/14

[1] Patients transfused with blood components.
[2] Patient misidentification at blood transfusion.

Complications of surgery

Five out of 12 patients (42%) undergoing a re-exploration subsequently died. Of the total mortality, 19% was observed in reoperated patients. In them, age, blood loss volume and number of red units transfused fell above the upper quartile of the overall patient distribution (Table 6.7). Also in deceased patients, age, blood loss volume and number of red units transfused fell above the upper quartile of the overall patient distribution.

The median LOS before surgery was four days (hinges: 2-8) and after surgery 11 days (hinges: 9-14). Although preoperative LOS did not differ among hospitals of the two broad geographic areas, five of seven with a median preoperative LOS higher than five days were in the Mediterranean area (Figure 6.30).

VI. Costs

Estimated costs per operated patient were ECU 395, partitioned according to the product as depicted in Figure 6.31.

Extremes belonging to the same geographic area were ECU 132 and 1 171. In the majority of the hospitals, red units were the product with more impact on the global costs; in a few hospitals, albumin and/or plasma were the products absorbing approximately half of the global costs (Figure 6.32).

Table 6.7. AAA: complications of surgery

	Reporting/all hospitals	Patient number	Age, years	Gender M:F	Preoperative Hct %	Perioperative bleeding, L	Postoperative bleeding, L	Red units per patient	Last Hct %	Postoperative LOS, days	Death day number after surgery
Reoperation for bleeding		12	74 (63-88)	11:1	40 (33-45)	3.6 (0.3-15.0)	. (1.0-6.0)	9 (3-32)	29 (17-44)	11 (0-43)	11 (0-41)
recorded in	7/23	12/693			10/12	9/12	3/12		9/12		5/12
deaths		26	75 (44-88)	5:1	41 (24-47)	2.4 (0.3-15.0)	1.6 (0.4-3.5)	8 (1-34)	30 (17-44)		7 (0-41)
recorded in	12/23	26/693			23/26	16/26	5/26	25/26	14/25		

¹ Median (range).
. = not calculated due to the small sample size.

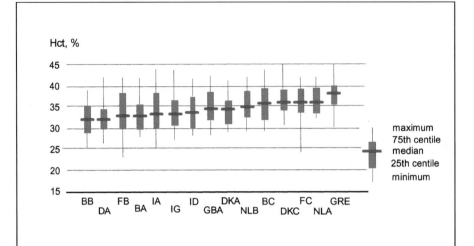

Fig 6.29. - AAA: last recorded Hct (after all transfusions have been given) in patients transfused with red units in each hospital. Each distribution refers to fifteen or more patients

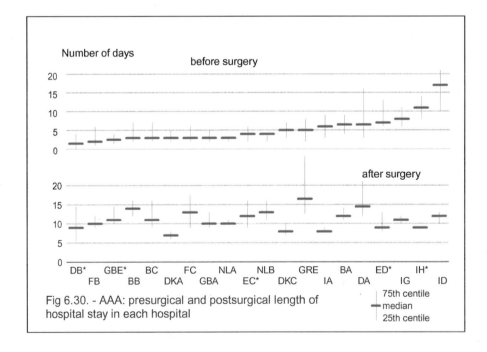

Fig 6.30. - AAA: presurgical and postsurgical length of hospital stay in each hospital

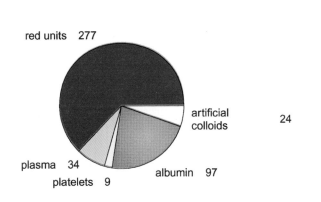

red units 277

artificial colloids 24

albumin 97

plasma 34

platelets 9

Fig 6.31. - AAA: estimated costs of the product used. Values indicate ECUs per patient operated

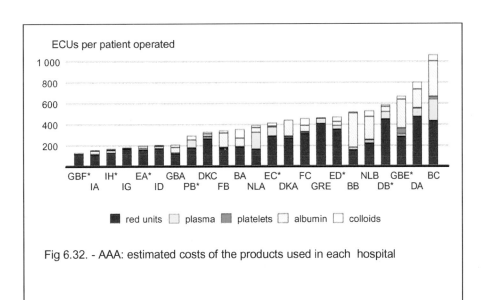

ECUs per patient operated

■ red units □ plasma ■ platelets □ albumin □ colloids

Fig 6.32. - AAA: estimated costs of the products used in each hospital

195

VII. Summary and comments on AAA

AAA patients received in decreasing proportions red units (83%), artificial colloids (64%), albumin (46%), plasma (26%) and platelets (3%). However, each of these proportions differed greatly among hospitals, even within a country: from 64 to 100% for red units, 0 to 100% for albumin, 0 to 100% for artificial colloids, 0 to 100% for plasma and 0 to 12% for platelets. Similar differences were also observed in the median amount of each product administered to recipients: from two to seven for red units, 0.5 to 1.9 L for artificial colloids, 26 to 122 g for albumin and one to eight units for plasma. In some hospitals (BC, DA, NLA), the more numerous the products used, the higher was the proportion of the recipients, and the larger the amount of product administered.

In perioperative red unit transfusion, some variables were found to affect both the proportion of transfused patients and the mean number of units. They included patient age and preoperative Hct, blood loss volumes and the use of autotransfusion. However, interhospital differences persisted after adjustment for age, preoperative Hct and blood loss. Different values attributed to these variables within each hospital in part explain the differences, but the hospital itself remains the major variable. Patient age was similar in hospitals included and not included in the analysis. Blood loss volumes and autotransfusion use were, however, higher and preoperative Hct values lower in hospitals which could not be analysed due to transfusion of nearly all patients.

The use of autotransfusion also varied among hospitals: the proportion of operated patients transfused with autologous units ranged from 0 to 85%. In hospitals of central-northern Europe it was half of that observed in hospitals of the Mediterranean area.

The threshold for transfusion of red units in the postoperative period was an Hct value of 27% ± 2.5.

The overall use of plasma was very high, with six hospitals transfusing the majority of the patients. One quarter of the patients received one or two units, a dose deemed ineffective in the treatment of coagulation disorders. No relevant information on patients is available; however, the reasons documented in the clinical records of some of the recipients indicate that plasma transfusions were given due to the occurrence of bleeding and for volume replacement. The reconstitution of whole blood by transfusing red blood cell concentrates and plasma accounted for 85% of plasma recipients. The use of liquid plasma, often observed in all surgical procedures in hospitals PB and NLA, is even more difficult to justify in hospitals where other effective, less risky and cheaper colloids are available.

Hospitals differed in the use of colloids according to a geographic pattern: in hospitals of central-northern Europe, the proportion of albumin recipients was 10 times higher than that observed in the Mediterranean area, and that of artificial colloids three times higher. Part of such diversities may be explained by a different access to the products in some countries. However, diversities from hospital to hospital were observed in both the proportion of recipients and amount given even within a country where the organization is expected to be homogeneous. Preferences play a great part in the differences, since, as already mentioned for other surgical procedures, the choice of fluid for volume replacement is still controversial and unsupported by proof of superior efficacy of any type of product. [16-21]

196

In some hospitals, albumin was not used as an alternative, but was additional to that of other colloids. Although information on patient comorbidity was not available, the observed frequency of albumin use does not seem to encompass the few indications at present available. [17,19]

Artificial colloids were used in all hospitals, with the exception of hospital DKA, where no artificial colloid was used in any of the six surveyed surgical procedures.

Final comments

The present study is the first Europe-wide survey on the use of blood products and artificial colloids in elective surgery. The results might reasonably be expected to be representative of the best practice since the study involved only large teaching hospitals that were willing to provide data.

The most striking finding is the wide variation among hospitals in the use of each of the studied products for similar categories of patients. These differences were also found among hospitals in the same country, where the organization of health care and the access to products might be expected to be homogeneous. Large differences in practice were also observed when we compared hospitals in the two broad geographic areas of Europe. In central-northern Europe, the use of albumin and artificial colloids was much greater while autotransfusion was more widely employed in hospitals in the Mediterranean countries.

Some variables, such as age, gender, preoperative Hct and blood loss, proved to influence the proportion of patients perioperatively transfused with red units. However, major hospital-to-hospital differences persisted after adjustment for these variables. Other factors, therefore, appear to have a powerful effect on the transfusion practice in the individual hospitals.

A similar variability in blood use has been reported in previous studies. [2-4] Some authors have suggested that major variables contributing to interhospital variation include: (a) ill-defined criteria for transfusion due to incomplete scientific knowledge; [11,12,23,24] (b) a lack of effective methods to consistently translate the available knowledge into clinical practice; [25,26] (c) differences in application of the criteria for transfusion [11,24] or differences in physicians' belief about the value of practices for meeting patient needs; [27] a negative association was found between knowledge and years of practice; [28] (d) an 'institutional' effect on transfusion practice (in CABG). [2]

The high use of whole blood rather than red cell concentrates in the hospitals of Great Britain and Greece was surprising. However, it is notable that in hospitals where whole blood was not used, red cell concentrates and plasma were often used together, effectively reconstituting whole blood. This practice clearly negates the widely accepted concept of blood component therapy and effectively doubles the risk to the patient for no provable benefit. Furthermore, in some hospitals plasma was used for volume replacement (as explicitly documented in the clinical record or suggested by the use of liquid plasma, since this product is not an effective source of labile coagulation factors). This clinical use of plasma unnecessarily exposes the patient to the virological risks of a blood component that is not virus-inactivated. It also diverts plasma that could otherwise be fractionated and also reduces the ability of European countries to achieve self-sufficiency in blood products using voluntary, unremunerated donors. [1]

A further wastage occurs in the practice of autotransfusion. Not only was PABD used in some hospitals for interventions (CHOLE, TURP) for which blood transfusion is very rarely needed, [13,14] but in only a few of the hospitals performing CABG, AAA and THR was the use of autotransfusion associated with a substantial reduction in patients transfused with allogeneic red units or in the number of allogeneic red units given to each patient. In hospitals where autotransfusion is frequently used, the transfusion of patients with red units was found to be largely independent of preoperative Hct values or blood loss. This suggests that the indications for transfusing autologous red units are more liberal than for allogeneic transfusion. It may also be the case that autologous blood is given simply because it is available. [14,15] Other authors have identified this as one of the causes of the low cost-effectiveness of PABD. [29]

Data from the present study have been compared with published studies. While for CHOLE, COLE, TURP and AAA there are only a few reports, reflecting the experience of individual centres with a limited number of patients, in the case of CABG and THR results of large multicentre retrospective studies have been recently published. For THR, the percentage of patients transfused with red units in the present study was similar to that reported by Toy *et al.*, [5] and higher than that reported by Surgenor *et al.*, [4] the latter finding a smaller variation among hospitals. For CABG, the percentage of transfused patients in the present study was higher than that reported by others, [2,3] with similar interhospital variations.

The wide variations in the percentage of patients receiving albumin and colloids, as well as in the quantity and combination of products given per recipient in hospitals using these products, were not surprising, since the choice of fluid for the management of acute hypovolaemia remains controversial and unsupported by proof of superior efficacy of any type of product. [16-21]

Among the outcomes assessed by Sanguis, haemolytic reactions were reported by only three out of 43 hospitals; it is not known whether there was under-reporting in the remaining hospitals.

The last Hct value before discharge was either below or above the range usually considered optimal (24 to 33%, [12]) in 0.3 to 0.7% and 43 to 64% of transfused patients, respectively. Since undertransfusion or no transfusion can put some patient categories at risk, the proportion of surgical patients leaving the hospital with Hct values below 24% should be monitored, especially since the increase in litigation over transfusion complications might increase the proportion of undertransfused patients. Conversely, overtransfusion implies wastage of limited donor resources, additional costs and needless risks for patients, including blood transmissible diseases and incompatible transfusion.

In most hospitals either a T&S or a blood request was routinely submitted for all patients undergoing either CHOLE or TURP. This is despite the fact that only 4 and 16%, respectively, of operated patients were ultimately transfused and only approximately half of them required transfusion according to accepted criteria. [11-12] While in particular conditions a T&S request cannot be avoided, the proximity of an effective transfusion service should discourage routine preoperative requests for blood or laboratory pretransfusion tests for these procedures.

Proper documentation is needed to ensure continuity of care, to allow for review of the possible causes of adverse events and to respond to medico-legal or clinical audit actions. In more than three quarters of patients transfused perioperatively with red units, no clinician's note was found indicating why transfusion was given (or specifying circumstances in which it was to be given).

In 53% of the hospitals the clinical record and the transfusion service records of recipients of allogeneic blood did not fully correspond. Furthermore, in only about one quarter of the hospitals was there documentation of any errors or adverse clinical events in transfusion. These problems are common, and failure to document them points either to a lack of appreciation of the implications for safety and accountability or perhaps to a reluctance to make a written record that may place the staff at risk of censure or possible legal action.

199

Taken altogether, the data from the Sanguis study indicate that the publication of consensus conference reports and guidelines on the use of blood in surgery has so far had a limited impact on transfusion practice in many clinical units, including those in teaching environments. Studies carried out in the hospital where the Sanguis project originated [9] demonstrated that improvement in the use of blood products can be achieved through an audit process based on simple indicators, providing the responsible clinicians with continuous feedback of results obtained. In a three-year period, this audit programme reduced both excessive preoperative requesting and actual transfusion of red units and plasma in elective surgical patients by 22, 20, and 70%, respectively. [10] Continuous feedback of data in laboratory medicine has been shown to reduce excessive ordering of laboratory tests [30] and other resources. [31] But other studies emphasize that intensive 'marketing' of accepted practice guidelines is required to produce changes in clinical practice. [32] The indicators referred to [9,10] as suitable for the identification of unnecessary preoperative blood ordering and avoidable transfusion of red units and plasma, have also proved useful in the present study. Data from Sanguis also point to the need for indicators to express the use of whole blood and albumin. In addition, undertransfusion should be revealed by monitoring the proportion of patients leaving hospital with an Hct below 24%. Simple indicators of the quality of documentation also seem to be needed. A cost evaluation should be made of a programme of audit, using these simple indicators, comparing the cost with the value of achieved improvements in quality of patient care, conservation of donor resources and financial savings.

References

[1] (a) Council of Europe. *Plasma products and European self-sufficiency: collection, preparation and use*, ISBN 92-871-1925-2, Strasbourg (France), Council of Europe Press, 1992.

(b) Commission of the European Communities. *Blood self-sufficiency in the European Community*, ISBN 92-77-55673-0, Luxembourg, Office for Official Publications of the European Communities, 1993.

(c) Council of Europe. *Responsibilities of health authorities in the field of blood transfusion*, Recommendation No R (88) 4, 1988 ISBN 92-871-1688-1, Council of Europe, Strasbourg (France), 1989.

(d) Council of Europe. Council Directive 89/381/EEC, *Official Journal of the European Communities*, L 181/46, 23.6.1989.

(e) European Parliament. Joint motion for a resolution on safe blood transfusions and the use of blood derivatives, 17 November 1993.

[2] Goodnough, L. T., Johnston, M. F. M., Toy, P. T. C. Y. and the Transfusion Medicine Academic Award Group. 'The variability of transfusion practice in coronary artery bypass surgery', *Journal of the American Medical Association*, 1991, 265: pp. 86-90.

[3] Surgenor, D. M., Wallace, E. L., Churchill, W. H. *et al.* 'Red cell transfusions in coronary artery bypass surgery (DRGs 106 and 107)'. *Transfusion*, 1992, 32: pp. 458-64.

[4] Surgenor, D. M., Wallace, E. L., Churchill, W. H. *et al.* 'Red cell transfusions in total knee and total hip replacement surgery', *Transfusion*, 1991, 31: pp. 531-37.

[5] Toy, P. T. C. Y., Kaplan, E. B., McVay, P. A. *et al.* 'Blood loss and replacement in total hip arthroplasty: a multicenter study', *Transfusion*, 1992, 32: pp. 63-67.

[6] Committee on autologous transfusion. 'Formula for standardizing the term salvaged unit of blood', *AABB News Briefs*, 1986, 9:6.

[7] Goodnight, J. H., Harvey, V. R. 'Least squares means in the fixed effects general model', SAS technical report R-103, 1978, SAS Institute, Cary, NC.

[8] Kleinbaum, D. G., Kupper, L. L., Morgenstern, H. *Epidemiologic research: principle and quantitative methods*, Belmont, CA, Wadsworth Inc., 1982.

[9] Giovanetti, A. M., Parravicini, A., Baroni, L. *et al.* 'Quality assessment of transfusion practice in elective surgery, *Transfusion*, 1988, 28: pp. 166-69.

[10] Giovanetti, A. M., Parravicini, A., Riccardi, D. *et al.* 'A quality improvement program of surgical blood transfusion practice', Symposium on blood conservation and surgery, Brussels (Belgium), 1 to 2 December 1989, Abstract book, p. 30.

[11] Welch, G. H., Meehan, K. R., Goodnough, L. T. 'Prudent strategies for elective red blood cell transfusion', *Annals of Internal Medicine*, 1992, 116: pp. 393-402.

[12] (a) Consensus Conference. 'Perioperative red cell transfusion', *Journal of the American Medical Association*, 1988, 260: pp. 2700-2703.

(b) Consensus Conference. National Institutes of Health. 'Platelet transfusion therapy', *Journal of the American Medical Association*, 1987, 257: pp. 177-80.

(c) Consensus Conference. National Institutes of Health. 'Fresh frozen plasma. Indications and risks', *Journal of the American Medical Association*, 1985, 253: pp. 551-6.

[13] Goodnough, L. T., Saha, P., Hirschler, N. V. *et al.* 'Autologous blood donation in nonorthopaedic surgical procedures as a blood conservation strategy', *Vox Sanguinis*, 1992, 63: pp. 96-101.

[14] The National Blood Resource Education Program Expert Panel. 'The use of autologous blood', *Journal of the American Medical Association*, 1990, 263: pp. 414-17.

[15] Kruskall, M. 'On measuring the success of an autologous blood donation program', *Transfusion*, 1991, 31: pp. 481-82.

[16] Fischer, M. McD. 'The crystalloid versus colloid controversy: bias, logic and toss-up', *Theoretical Surgery*, 1989, 4: pp. 205-11.

[17] Durand-Zaleski, I., Bonnet, F., Rochant, H. *et al.* 'Usefulness of consensus conferences: the case of albumin, *The Lancet*, 1992, 340: 1388-90.

[18] Messmer, K. F. W. 'The use of plasma substitutes with special attention to their side effects'. *World Journal of Surgery*, 1987, 11: pp. 69-74.

[19] Erstad. B. L., Gales, B. J., Rappaport, W. D. 'The use of albumin in clinical practice', *Archives of Internal Medicine*, 1991, 151: pp. 901-11.

[20] Stockwell, M. A., Soni, N., Riley, B. 'Colloid solutions in the critically ill. A randomised comparison of albumin and polygeline. 1. Outcome and duration of stay in the intensive care unit', *Anaesthesia*, 1992, 47: pp. 3-6.

[21] Stockwell, M. A., Scott, A., Day, A., Riley, B., Soni, N. 'Colloid solutions in the critically ill. A randomised comparison of albumin and polygeline. 2. Serum albumin concentration and incidences of pulmonary oedema and acute renal failure' *Anaesthesia*, 1992, 47: pp. 7-9.

[22] Rawle, P. R., Seeley, H. F. 'Assessing blood volume, blood loss and blood replacement', *British Journal of Hospital Medicine*, 1987, 38: pp. 554-7.

[23] Levine, E., Rosen, A., Sehgal, L., *et al.* 'Physiologic effects of acute anemia: implications for a reduced transfusion trigger', *Transfusion*, 1990, 30: pp. 11-14.

[24] Carson, J. L., Rees Willett, L. 'Is hemoglobin of 10 g/dL required for surgery?', *Medical Clinics of North America*, 1993, 2: pp. 335-47.

[25] Linton, A. L., Peachey, D. K. 'Guidelines for medical practice: the reasons why', *Canadian Medical Association Journal*, 1990, 143: pp. 485-90.

[26] Berwick, D. M., Enthoven, A., Bunker, J.P. 'Quality management: the doctor's role-I', *British Medical Journal* 1992, 304: pp. 235-38.

[27] Mulley, A. G., Eagle, K. A. 'What is inappropriate care?', *Journal of the American Medical Association*, 1988, 260: pp. 540-41.

[28] Salem-Schatz, S. R., Avorn, J., Sourmerai, S.B. 'Influence of clinical knowledge, organizational context and practice style on transfusion decision making. Implications for practice change strategies', *Journal of the American Medical Association*, 1990, 264: pp. 471-75.

[29] Birkmeyer, J. D., Goodnough, L. T., AuBouchon, L. T. *et al.* 'The cost-effectiveness of preoperative blood donation for total hip and knee replacement', *Transfusion*, 1993, 33: pp. 544-51.

[30] Studnicki, J., Bradham, D. D., Marshburn, J., Foulis, P. R., Straumfjord, J. V. A feedback system for reducing excessive laboratory tests', *Archives of Pathology and Laboratory Medicine*, 1993, 117: pp. 35-39.

[31] Russell, I., Grimshaw, J. 'The effectiveness of referral guidelines: a review of the methods and findings of published evaluations', Chapter 13, in: Roland, M., Coulder, A. (Eds): *Hospital referrals*, Oxford General Practice Series No 22, 1992, pp. 179-211.

[32] Lomas, J., Enkin, M., Anderson, G. M., Hannah, W. J., Vayda, E. 'Opinion leaders vs audit and feedback to implement practice guidelines. Delivery after previous cesarean section', *Journal of the American Medical Association*, 1991, 265: pp. 2202-7.

Most of the information reported in the box under the title of each surgical procedure was taken from Sabiston. D. C. (Ed). *Textbook of surgery. The biologic basis of modern surgery*, Philadelphia, USA W. B. Saunders Publishers, 1991.

Acknowledgements

This study would have not been possible without the cooperation of clinical staff in all the participating hospitals and the enthusiastic participation of the data collectors.

Contributions from local institutions raised by national coordinators have made the completion of the Sanguis study possible.

Glossary of abbreviations

The following abbreviations, notations and conventions were used in the text, figures and tables:

Albumin	different concentrations and volumes were transformed into grams of albumin
Allogeneic	human blood from a genetically unrelated donor
Artificial colloids	gelatins, dextrans, hydroxy-aminoethyl starch (HES)
Autologous blood	the patient's own blood, collected by one or several techniques (e.g. PABD, PIH, IBS), so that it can be reinfused during or after operation
Autotransfusion	the reinfusion of autologous blood
Blood components	whole blood, red cell concentrates, plasma, platelets, cryoprecipitates
Blood products	blood components and plasma fractions
Case report form	*ad hoc* form in which all clinical and transfusion events occurring in each patient are recorded in accordance with the protocol of the study
DVT	deep venous thrombosis
g	gram
Hct	haematocrit
Hinges	25th and 75th centile of the distribution of a variable
Hospital code	code of the country (one or two letters) followed by a letter
Hospital code*	hospital with a patient number lower than 20
IBS	intraoperative autologous transfusion (intraoperative blood salvage). Salvaged units were transformed into corresponding red blood cell concentrates by applying a published formula [6]
L	litre
Last Hct	the one recorded closest to the day of discharge; in patients transfused with red units it represented the one recorded after all transfusions had been given
LOS	length of hospital stay
MSBOS	maximum surgical blood order schedule. A list of surgical procedures indicating the type of preoperative request and the number of red units to be requested preoperatively. Usually part of hospital standard procedures
M:F	male to female ratio
MR	in-hospital crude mortality rate, expressed as percent of operated patients
NSAID	non steroidal anti-inflammatory drugs
NOS	not otherwise specified
PABD	preoperative autologous blood donation
Perioperative	from the day of surgery to three days after, included
PIH	preoperative isovolaemic haemodilution
Plasma	liquid and fresh frozen plasma, obtained from whole blood donation and by apheresis, and unless otherwise specified, both autologous and allogeneic. Plasma units obtained from apheresis were by convention counted as equivalent to two units of units obtained from standard donation
Plasma fractions	albumin 5% or 20% and any other therapeutic product prepared from human plasma under pharmaceutical manufacturing conditions
Platelets	platelet concentrate, obtained from whole blood donation or by apheresis. Platelets obtained by apheresis were conventionally made equal to five units of those obtained from the standard donation
Postoperative	from the fourth day after surgery to the day of discharge from hospital
Preoperative	from the day of hospital admission to the day before intervention

Products	blood components, albumin, artificial colloids
Red units	red blood cell concentrates or whole blood units, and unless otherwise specified both autologous and allogeneic
Request	a request for blood components or for Type and Screen (T&S) made before and for the intervention
Reoperation	percentage of operated patients who underwent a revision for bleeding during the hospital stay
Transfusion episode	transfusions given within a calendar day
Type and Screen	a procedure of the transfusion service: pretransfusion tests are performed on the patient blood sample, no red units are reserved for the patient, and a simplified compatibility test between donor and recipient is performed should blood be released
Use of products	expressed mainly by:

   (i) percentage of operated patients who were transfused with a given product;

   (ii) percentage of transfused patients according to a variable (e.g. time of transfusion);

   (iii) number of units (g for albumin, L for colloids) per patient transfused, mean $\pm$ SD, median, hinges, and range;

   (iv) number of units (g for albumin, L colloids) per patient operated, mean, median and hinges.

Data collectors

Dr D. Almini
Centro Trasfusionale e di Immunologia dei Trapianti, Ospedale Maggiore, I - Milano

Dr V. Apostolopoulou
Asklepion Orthopaedic Hospital, GR - Athens

Dr K. Bell
Department of Transfusion Medicine, Royal Infirmary of Edinburgh, UK - Edinburgh

Mrs B. Borregaard
Universitetshospital, Skejby Sygehus, DK - Aarhus

Dr J. Brook
Welsh Regional Transfusion Centre, Rhydlafar, UK - Cardiff

Dr P. Chiavolini
Servizio Trasfusionale, USSL 28 Legnago, I - Legnago

Dr M. Chin Tad Muon
Serviço de Imunohemoterapia, Hospitais da Universidade de Coimbra, P - Coimbra Codex

Dr M. T. Colotti
Centro Trasfusionale e di Immunologia, Istituto Ortopedico G. Pini, I - Milano

Dr J. Diaz
Servicios Hemoterapia, Hospital de la Santa Creu i Sant Pau, E - Barcelona

Dr G. Gandini
Servizio Trasfusionale Istituti Ospitalieri - USSL 25, I - Verona

Dr I. Gentilini
Centro Trasfusionale, Ospedale Generale Regionale, I - Bolzano

Dr N. Georgakopoulos
General Regional University Hospital, GR - Rion-Patras

Dr M. Girard
Centre National de Transfusion Sanguine, Etablissement Saint-Antoine, F - Paris Cedex 12

Dr S. Gray
Department of Transfusion Medicine, Royal Infirmary of Edinburgh, UK - Edinburgh

Dr G. Graziani
Servizio Trasfusionale, Ospedale Policlinico Careggi, I - Firenze

Dr H. Hansen
Righospitalet, DK - Copenhagen

Dr W. E. Hitzler
Blutbank, Chirurgische Klinik der Universität Heidelberg, D - Heidelberg

Dr J. M. Hurpé
Département d'Anesthésie Réanimation Chirurgicale, CHRU de Caen, F - Caen Cedex

Dr J. Jimenez
Banco de Sangre, Hospital Clinique, E - Barcelona

Miss D. McLoughlin
Regional Blood Transfusion Service, UK - Sheffield

Dr K. Makris
Transfusion Service, Trauma Hospital (KAT), GR - Athens

Dr J. Manel
Département d'Anesthésie-Réanimation, CHU, F - Nancy Cedex

Mrs I. Möller
Universitetshospital, Skejby Sygehus, DK - Aarhus

Dr D. Olzer
Servizio Trasfusionale, Istituti Ospitalieri - USSL 25, I - Verona

Dr R. C. Pereira
Serviço de Imunohemoterapia, Hospital de S. Joao, P - Porto

Dr J. Roldan
Hospital de la Santa Creu i Sant Pau, E - Barcelona

Dr T. Rosenberg
Department of Surgery, Laikon General Hospital, GR - Athens

Dr C. Sacchi
Servizio di Anestesiologia, Istituto Ortopedico 'R. Galeazzi', I - Milano;

Dr C. Sanchez
Transfusion Service, Princeps d'Espagna, L'Hospital de Llobregat, E - Madrid

Dr B. Sloth Christiansen
Aalborg Sygehus, DK - Aalborg

Dr S. Solinas
Centro Trasfusionale, Università degli Studi 'La Sapienza', I - Roma

Dr J. Spiliotopoulou
1st Regional Transfusion Center, Hippokrateion Hospital, GR - Athens

Dr Theodosiadis
1st Regional Transfusion Center, Hippokrateion Hospital, GR - Athens

Dr R. Toscano
Banco de Sangre, Hospital 12 de Octubre, E - Madrid

Dr K. C. van Dalen
Academisch Ziekenhuis, NL - Groningen

Dr H. Vouga
Laboratory of Haematology and Transfusion Medicine, University of Patras Medical School, GR - Patras

Mrs H. Waterloos
Cliniques Universitaires Saint-Luc, B - Brussels

Dr C. Weiß
Abt für Experimentelle Chirurgie, Klinikum der Universität Heidelberg, D - Heidelberg

Data managing

Roberta Maserati, ScD
Centro Trasfusionale e di Immunologia dei Trapianti, Ospedale Maggiore, I - Milan

Data processing

Mr Gaetano Caltagirone, W Bergamaschi, ScD
Centro Trasfusionale e di Immunologia dei Trapianti, Ospedale Maggiore, I - Milan

Participating hospitals and clinicians

Belgium
Academisch Ziekenhuis, VUB, Brussels
(Dr L. Steensens, Dr J. Flament, Dienst Hematologie)

Clinique Universitaires Saint-Luc, UCL, Brussels
(Prof. M. De Bruyere, Centre de Transfusion Sanguine)

Hôpital Erasme, ULB, Brussels
(Dr M. Lambermont, Prof. E. Dupont), Centre d'Immuno-Hematologie et Transfusion Sanguine)

Denmark
Aalborg Hospital, Aalborg
(Dr C. Jersild, Regional Blood Transfusion Service)

Rigshospitalet, Copenhagen
(Dr H. Soerensen, Blood Transfusion Service)

University Hospital, Aarhus
(Dr J. Joergensen, Blood Transfusion Service)

France
CHRU Hôpital Central, Nancy-Cédex
(Prof. M. C. Laxenaire, Départment d'Anesthésie-Réanimation; Dr F. Streiff, Centre Régional de Transfusion Sanguine)

CHRU, Grenoble-Cédex
(Prof. P. Girardet, Département d'Anesthésie-Réanimation; Prof. P. Magnin, Centre Régional de Transfusion Sanguine)

CHRU, Caen-Cédex
(Prof. H. Bricard, Département d'Anesthésie-Réanimation; Prof. M. Thomas, Centre Régional de Transfusion Sanguine)

Hôpital Saint-Antoine, Paris Cédex 12
(Prof. A. Lienhart, Départment d'Anesthésie-Réanimation, Dr M. Girard, Centre Régional de Transfusion Sanguine)

Germany
Klinikum der Universität Heidelberg, Chirurgische Klinik, Heidelberg
(Dr W. E. Hitzler, Blutbank)

Klinikum Grosshadern d. Ludwig-Maximilians, Universität, Munich
(Prof. W. Mempel, Dr M. Schwarzfisher, Transfusionszentrum; Dr M. Haller, Institut für Anesthesiologie; Dr M. Schmöckl, Dr G. Nollert, Herzchirurgische Klinik; Dr M. Heiss, Dr M. Kirschner, Chirurgische Klinik; Dr M. Kriegmair, Klinik für Urologie; Dr T. Pfeifer, Klinik für Orthopädie)

United Kingdom
Deaconess Hospital, Edinburgh
(Dr D. B. L. McClelland, Regional Blood Transfusion Service)

King Edward IV Hospital, Sheffield
(Dr W. Wagstaff, Regional Blood Transfusion Service)

Northern General Hospital, Sheffield
(Dr W. Wagstaff, Regional Blood Transfusion Service)

Prince of Wales Hospital, Cardiff
(Dr J. Napier, National Blood Transfusion Service, Welsh Regional Transfusion Centre)

Princess Margaret Rose Orthopaedic Hospital, Edinburgh
(Dr D. B. L. McClelland, Regional Blood Transfusion Service)

Royal Infirmary, Edinburgh
(Dr D. B. L. McClelland, Regional Blood Transfusion Service)

Royal Hallamshire Hospital, Sheffield
(Dr W. Wagstaff, Regional Blood Transfusion Service)

University Hospital, Cardiff
(Dr J. Napier, National Blood Transfusion Service, Welsh Regional Transfusion Centre)

Western General Hospital, Edinburgh
(Dr D. B. L. McClelland, Regional Blood Transfusion Service)

Greece

Asklepion Orthopaedic, Athens
(Dr O. Marantidou, Blood Transfusion Service)

Greek Anticancer Institute, Athens
(Dr M. Moraki, Blood Transfusion Service)

Hippokrateion Hospital, Athens
(Dr I. Kantopoulou, First Regional Transfusion Center)

Laikon General Hospital, Athens
(Dr T. Mandalaki, Blood Transfusion Service)

Regional University Hospital, Patras
(Prof. A. Maniatis, Dr H. Theodoris, Blood Transfusion Service)

Trauma Hospital (KAT), Athens
(Dr A. Axenidou, Blood Transfusion Service)

Italy

Istituti Ospitalieri, Verona
(Dr G. Aprili, Servizio Trasfusionale)

Istituto Ortopedico G Galeazzi, Milano
(Prof. G. Oriani, Reparto di Anestesia e Rianimazione)

Istituto Ortopedico G Pini, Milano
(Dr F. Mercuriali, Centro Trasfusionale)

Ospedale Generale Regionale, Bolzano
(Dr O. Prinoth, Servizio Trasfusionale)

Ospedale Maggiore, Milano
(Dr M. Langer, Prof. G. Japichino, Reparto di Anestesia e Rianimazione)

Ospedale Policlinico Universitario di Careggi, Firenze
(Dr G. Avanzi, Centro Trasfusionale)

Ospedale Provinciale di Legnago, Legnago
(Dr A. Disperati, Servizio Trasfusionale)

Università degli Studi La Sapienza, Roma
(Prof G. Isacchi, Centro Trasfusionale)

Portugal

Hospitais da Universidade de Coimbra, Coimbra Codex
(Prof. R. B. Carrington da Costa, Unidade de Cuidados Intensivos)

Hospital de San Joao, Porto

Spain
Hospital de la Santa Creu i Sant Pau, Barcelona
(Dr I. Casas, Servicio de Anestesia y Reanimaciòn; Dr R. Suñol, Mrs L. Martin, Department of Quality Assurance)

Hospital Princeps d'Espanya, L'Hospital de Llobregat
(Dr C. Ferran, Hematology Service and Blood Bank)

Hospital Clinic, Barcelona
(Dr R. Castillo, Servicio de Hemoterapia)

Hospital 12 de Octubre, Madrid
(Dr J. Montero, Servizio de Hemotherapia)

The Netherlands
Academisch Ziekenhuis, Groningen
(Dr C. Smit Sibinga, Bloedbank)

Roman Catholic Hospital, Groningen
(Dr C. Smit Sibinga, Bloedbank)

Appendices

Appendix 1
Protocol for data collection

PROTOCOL FOR DATA COLLECTION

IV Version
December 1990

CODING:

Surgical unit   [_ _ _] Hospital   [_ _]

Hospital Transfusion Service   [_ _] Cumulative   [_ _ _ _ _ _]

PART I: PATIENT DATA collected in the SURGICAL UNIT

1.0. Patient identification number (ID code) ....
      Patient last, first name ....
      Case No.(progressive) ....
      Sex M F   birthdate   .. / .. / .. (day.month.year)

2.0. Hospital stay: date of admission   .. / .. / ..
                                    date of discharge   .. / .. / ..
                                    date of death   .. / .. / ..
                                    date of operation   .. / .. / ..

3.0. Preoperative diagnosis
      cholelithiasis   []   colorectal cancer   []
      prostate adenoma   []   coronary artery disease   []
      abdominal aortic aneurysm   []   hip arthrosis deformans   []

4.0. Drug administration no []   yes []
                                    preoperative   intraoperative   postoperative
                                    (within 7 days)

      aspirine and non steroid
      anti-inflammatory drugs (NSAID) []
      desmopressin   []   []
      heparin (low dose)   []   []
      heparin (anticoagulant dose)   []   []
      aprotinin   []   []
      tranexamic acid   []   []
      coumarin   []
      EACA   []   []

5.0. Surgical procedure performed
      cholecystectomy: laparotomic   []   laparoscopic []
      colectomy: partial   []   subtotal   []
                          abdomino-perineal colorectal amputation []
      prostatectomy: transurethral (TURP) []   open   []
      coronary artery bypass graft (CABG):
                          with extracorporeal circulation   []
                          without extracorporeal circulation   []
                          mammary graft   []   saphenous graft   []
                          mammary & saphenous graft []   other graft   []
      abdominal aorta aneurysmectomy (AAA):
                          aortobi-femoral graft []
                          aortobi-iliac graft   []
                          aorto-aortic T-T graft []
      total hip replacement (THR)   []
      5.1.   duration of operation: ....

6.0. Anesthesia: general []   regional []   combined []

7.0. Estimated blood loss not recorded []   recorded [], if so:
      intraoperative .... ml   total postoperative .... ml

217

8.0. **Autologous blood procured**   no []   yes []:
number of units predeposited ....   salvaged ....   by hemodilution ....

9.0. **Preoperative blood request (for surgery)** no []   yes []   date ../../..

     9.1.   number of blood units requested

	predeposited	homologous
whole blood	...	...
red blood cell concentrate	...	...
fresh frozen plasma	...	...
liquid plasma	...	...
lyophilized plasma		...
platelets		...
cryoprecipitate		...

     9.2.   request of Type and Screen []

10.0. Data available in patient records

days   ------------>

	admission	preoperative				0	perioperative			postoperative				discharge
		-..	-3	-2	-1	0	+1	+2	+3	+4	+5	+..	+..	
DATE						sur-gery								
10.1 Hct (%) Hb/dL lowest daily value						@								

10.2.   Blood components transfused, number of units:

		admission													discharge
WHOLE BLOOD	homologous predeposited hemodilution salvaged @@														
RBCs	homologous predeposited salvaged														
FFP	homologous - standard don. - apheresis predeposited														
PLT	- standard don - apheresis														
Liquid plasma															
Cryoprecipitate															

@ following hemodilution (only in patients submitted to the procedure)   @@ without washing cycle

218

admission	days -------> preoperative				perioperative				postoperative				discharge
	- ..	- 3	- 2	- 1	0	+ 1	+ 2	- 3	- 4	+ 5	+ ..	+ ..	
DATE					sur-gery								

10.3.   Blood derivatives transfused

Albumin	(ml)													
	conc.(%)													
Lyophil.plasma	(ml)													
	conc.(%)													

10.4.   Artificial colloids (ml)

Gelatine:													
Urea-linked	3.5%												
Modif. fluid	4.0%												
Oxypolygelat.	5.5%												
Dextran 40	3.5%												
Dextran 40	10%												
Dextran 60	6%												
Dextran 70	6%												
HES 450/0.7	6%												
HES 200/0.5	6%												
HES 200/0.5	10%												
HES 200/0.62	6%												
HES 40/0.5	6%												

11.0.   Stated reason for transfusion available in patient records   no [ ]   yes [ ]
Perioperative period only

	anemia Hct%= ..	volume replacement	bleeding	laboratory coag. abnormality @	other
Whole blood					
RBCs					
FFP					
Liq./lyoph. plasma					
Cryoprecipitate					
PLT					
Albumin					
Artificial colloids					

@ coagulation tests: PT (%) ...   PTT (sec.) ...   PLTS (x10 exp.9/L) ...
Fibrinogen (mg/dL) ...   FDP (ug/dL) ...   TCT (sec.) ...

219

12.0. Complications during hospital stay available in patient records

no [] yes []

12.1. of surgery   [] :

reoperation for bleeding   []

12.2. of homologous blood transfusion   []

hemolytic reaction   []

fever/rigors   []

skin reaction   []

problems in blood administration:

patient misidentification at blood sample withdrawal   []

patient misidentification at blood transfusion   []

laboratory mismatch   []

12.3. of autotransfusion   []

12.3.1. at the donation   []

anemia   []   Hct (%) <..

fainting   []

seizure   []

bradycardia   []

tachycardia   []

other   []   ....(specify)

12.3.2 at the transfusion   []

hemolytic reaction   []

fever/rigors   []

skin reaction   []

problems in blood administration:

patient misidentification at blood sample withdrawal   []

patient misidentification at blood transfusion   []

laboratory mismatch   []

homologous blood given when autologous blood was available []

The above data have been collected by

name ....

address ....

telephone No. ....   Fax No. ....

Copy of these data have been sent also to

....

....

Note ....

....

date   .. / .. / ..

CODING:
Transfusion Service [_]   Hospital   [_ _]
Surgical Unit   [_ _ _]   Cumulative   [_ _ _ _ _ _ _]

PART II: PATIENT DATA collected in the TRANSFUSION SERVICE

1.0.   Patient ID (code) ....
       Last, first name ....
       sex M F   birthdate   . . / . . / . .

2.0.   Preoperative request to Transfusion Service (for surgery)   no [] yes []:
       2.1.   signed by: consultant   []   surgeon   []   anesthesiologist   []
                           nurse   []   medical student   []
                           unknown   []   other   []   ....(specify)
       2.2.   date of request. . / . . / . .
       2.3.   diagnosis   not stated   []   stated []
       2.4.   surgical procedure not stated   []   stated []   if so:
              cholecystectomy   [] :   laparotomic   []   laparoscopic   []
              colectomy :   partial   []   subtotal   []
                                           abdomino-perineal colorectal amputation   []
              prostatectomy   []:   transurethral (TURP) []   open   []
              coronary artery bypass graft (CABG):
                                           with extracorporeal circulation   []
                                           without extracorporeal circulation   []
              abdominal aorta aneurysmectomy repair (AAA)[]
              total hip replacement (THR)   []

       2.5.   Date of surgery   . . / . . / . .

       2.6.   hematocrit value   not stated   []   stated []   value ... %
       2.7.   No. of blood units requested   predeposited homologous
                     whole blood   ...   ...
                     red blood cell concentrate   ...   ...
                     fresh frozen plasma   ...   ...
                     liquid plasma   ...   ...
                     platelets   ...
                     cryoprecipitate   ...

       2.8.   Request according to MSBOS   no [] yes [] MSBOS not available []

       2.9.   Type and Screen   []   Crossmatch   [].

3.0.   Autologous blood procured :   no [] yes []
       number of units   predeposited   ....
                           salvaged   ....
                           by hemodilution ....

221

4.0. Blood units delivered and not returned   no [ ] yes [ ]

	days ------->												
admission	preoperative				perioperative				postoperative				discharge
	- ..	- 3	- 2	- 1	0	+ 1	+ 2	+ 3	+ 4	+ 5	+ .	+ ..	
DATE					sur-gery								

4.1.   Blood components, number of units:

WHOLE BLOOD	homologous predeposited hemodilution salvaged @@													
RBCs	homologous predeposited salvaged													
FFP	homologous - standard don. - apheresis predeposited													
PLT	- standard don - apheresis													
Liquid plasma														
Cryoprecipitate														

@ without washing cycle

5.0.   Complications during hospital stay reported or recorded
by the Transfusion Service   no [ ] yes [ ]
      5.1.   of homologous blood transfusion   [ ]
                hemolytic reaction   [ ]
                fever/rigors   [ ]
                skin reaction   [ ]
                problems in blood administration:
                patient misidentification at blood sample withdrawal   [ ]
                patient misidentification at blood transfusion   [ ]
                laboratory mismatch   [ ]
      5.2.   of autotransfusion [ ]
           5.2.1. at the donation   [ ]
                    anemia   [ ]   Hct (%) < ..
                    fainting   [ ]
                    seizure   [ ]
                    bradycardia   [ ]
                    tachycardia   [ ]
                    other   [ ] ....(specify)

5.2.2 <u>at the transfusion</u>   []
           hemolytic reaction   []
           fever/rigors   []
           skin reaction   []
           problems in blood administration:
           patient misidentification at blood sample withdrawal   []
           patient misidentification at blood transfusion   []
           laboratory mismatch   []
           homologous blood given when autologous blood was
           available   []

The above data have been collected by

name ....

address ....

telephone No. ....   Fax No. ....

Copy of these data have been sent also to

....
....

Note ....
....

date   .. / .. / ..

Appendix 2
Sanguis publication policy

Sanguis publication policy

The following policy has been established in order to guarantee an adequate and controlled flow of information on the Sanguis project and the results obtained within this project.

1. For all oral and written presentations of the concept and the results obtained within the Sanguis project, the written permission of the project leader (PL), Prof. Sirchia, I-Milano, is required.

2. This applies for international and national congresses and all publication media.

3. Permission from the PL has to be obtained prior to the submission of abstract/s, manuscript/s, and/or title/s for an oral presentation.

4. To obtain permission from the PL, a written application has to be submitted one month before to Prof. Sirchia with copies mailed at the same time to the members of the Project Management Group who will forward their remarks, if any, to the PL within seven days from receipt. In default of any notification, the PL will assume an approval.

5. The initial oral presentations on the concepts and the results of the Sanguis project to be given at international meeting will be by Dr McClelland, Prof. Messmer and Prof. Sirchia on behalf of all the participants.

6. The interim and final reports will be published by the Sanguis Study Group with a list of the names of all the participants on a footnote. The final report will be published in journals in the fields of transfusion medicine, surgery, anaesthesiology and general medicine, respectively.

7. In the publications of results obtained within Sanguis in one of the participating countries, all institutions and individuals involved in the data generation will be listed.

8. Sanguis has to be identified as a concerted action of the European Commission, IV Medical and Health Research Programme on the title of all publications.

Appendix 3
Consistency and coherence controls implemented in the computerized program

Consistency and coherence controls implemented in the computerized program

ITEM   MEANING

1. Consistency   reflecting a specified principle; free from internal contradiction
2. Coherence   the existence of a correlation between two or more specified data
3. Reliability   the amount of credence placed in a result

1. CONSISTENCY CONTROLS (Protocol Part I,II)

1.1. Formal controls

Entered = Expected (dates, numbers, Y/N, M/F)

1.2. Control of missing values (blanks)

Protocol Part I
Items controlled for blank, independently of other conditions:

sex	birthdate	admission date
discharge or death date	operation date	preoperative diagnosis
surgical procedure performed	drug administration	anaesthesia
blood loss recorded	autologous blood procured	preoperative blood request
complications of surgery		

Protocol Part II

If the patient is unknown to the Transfusion Service, Protocol Part II has to be ignored, therefore all the fields to be controlled for blank underlie other conditions.

1. If preoperative request = Y, control of blanks in the following items:

signed by	date of request	diagnosis stated
surgical procedure stated	date of surgery	haematocrit stated
blood units requested	MSBOS available	Type and Screen
crossmatch		

2. If the surgical procedure was stated on the request, the surgical procedure type has to be entered.

3. If the MSBOS was available, the question 'request according to MSBOS' has to be completed.

1.3. Control on coding (to verify if the codes entered are included in the related table)

Items controlled:
(i) preoperative diagnosis;
(ii) surgical procedure;
(iii) anaesthesia.

231

1.4. Consistency of dates

Date of:
1900 ≤ birth ≤ 1977

admission, blood request, transfusions, lab tests = 1990 or 1991
surgery, discharge, death

1.5. Consistency of some items

ITEM	ACCEPTED VALUE		
Blood loss	>0;	≤99 999 mL	

No of blood units:

(i) predeposited	≥ − 1;	≤10	
(ii) salvaged	≥ − 1;	≤30	
(iii) by haemodilution	≥ − 1;	≤10	**Note**

Note
The convention is:
− 1 = value not known;
→ note that it is possible to
enter a value of '0', but this
is not correct in these fields

No of units of blood, blood components:

(i) requested preoperatively	≥ − 1;	≤30
(ii) transfused (daily)	≥ − 1;	≤30

Artificial colloids

Blood derivatives:

administered daily	≥ − 1;	≤99 999 mL

Laboratory tests:

Hct (%)	≥ 9.0;	≤	60.0 on line max Hct
Hb g/dL	≥ 2.5;	≤	20.0 on line min Hb
PT (%)	≥ 0;	≤	150
PTT (sec.)	≥15;	≤	240
PLTS (x10⁹/L)	≥ 0;	≤	2 000
Fibrinogen (mg/dL)	≥ 0;	≤	1 000
FDP (ug/dL)	≥ 0;	≤32 000	
TCT (sec.)	≥ 10;	≤	100

Duration of:

hospital stay	≤	60 days
surgery	≤	600 minutes

Abbreviations: PT = prothrombin time; PTT = partial thromboplastin time; PLTS = platelets; FDP = fibrinogen degradation products; TCT = thrombin clotting time; PT value to be given as a percentage, PTT and TCT as time (in seconds)

2. COHERENCE CONTROLS (PROTOCOL PART I, II)

2.1. Between dates

Date of:

birth < admission   ≤ surgery   ≤ discharge, death
                    ≤ transfusions   ≤ discharge, death

birth < blood request   not < 30 days from admission ≤ surgery
     < lab tests   not < 30 days from admission

2.2. Between N/Y answers

IF	THEN
the answer is N	the underlying items have to be blank
the answer is Y	at least one of the underlying items has to be filled

This control is implemented for:

1. all the N/Y answers implying the use of codes listed on the on-line tables;
2. 'autologous blood units procured' and the related fields 'number of units predeposited, salvaged, by haemodilution';
3. 'blood loss recorded' and the related fields 'intraoperative mL'; 'total postoperative mL'.

Note: Where the answer is Y but the value is not known, see note 1.5 above.

2.3. Between items

IF	THEN
1. a specified diagnosis	a related surgical procedure
2. an anwer Y in 'preoperative blood request-ed'	at least one of the related fields 'blood units requested' and 'T&S' has to be Y (protocol Part I)
3. an anwer not blank (= N or Y) in 'stated reason for transfusion' (of blood, blood components, derivatives, artificial colloids)	one or more transfusions (of blood, blood components, blood derivatives, artificial colloids, in the perioperative period)
4. the answer to the question 'stated reason for transfusion' is Y and 'laboratory coagulation abnormalities' is the option selected from the related table	the field 'coagulation tests' has to be filled, otherwise it has to be blank (ignored)
5. an answer not blank in 'complications of homologous blood transfusion'	one or more homologous blood units transfused
6. an answer not blank in 'complications of autotransfusion at donation'	one or more blood units predeposited or obtained by haemodilution
7. an answer not blank in 'complications of autotransfusion at the transfusion'	one or more autologous blood units transfused (or homologous, if given when autologous were available)

3. CONVENTIONS

As a general rule:

N: the answer to the question is NO (information was looked for and found to be negative); if the answer is NO, subsequent items of that question have to be ignored.

Y: the answer to the question is YES (information was looked for and found to be positive); if the answer is Yes, at least one of the subsequent items of that question has to be filled; the remaining items, if they are negative or unknown, have to be ignored.

Dates are expressed as: day.month.year.

Blood units and blood components: only integer values. For intraoperative blood salvaging, values expressed as mL have to be transformed in number of units (integer) by the data collector before entering the data: see enclosed AABB recommendation.

If the data collector could not find any record pertaining quantities, the negative number − 1 is to be entered in the program, to conventionally indicate not known in the following items:
 (i) number of blood units predeposited, salvaged, obtained by haemodilution;
 (ii) number of blood units, blood components requested preoperatively;
 (iii) number of blood units, blood components transfused daily;
 (iv) volume of blood derivatives and/or artificial colloids transfused daily.

Protocol Part I, II

Patient ID: it may be the one used in the hospital. It is also possible to use a code assigned by the data collector provided it acts as an identification code.
By entering patient ID number in Protocol Part II, the patient's name (if available in Part I), along with sex and birthdate, are automatically displayed. Every subsequent modification entered in these fields in Protocol Part II does not update Part I and vice versa. Incoherences in patient identification fields between Part I and Part II have to be avoided.
Should the patient not be known at the Transfusion Service, simply ignore Part II as a whole.

Birthdate: use 01.01.year, if day and month cannot be entered for confidential reasons.

Surgical procedure performed - Colectomy:
1. partial   = excision of a named anatomical segment, e.g. right, left, transverse or sigmoid; include operations recorded as Rt or Lt Hemicolectomy.
2. subtotal = whole colon removed and rectum retained.
3. abdomino-perineal colorectal amputation = residual if both colon and rectum.

Duration of operation = ignore this field if the information is not known (facultative field).

Date of surgery has to be entered in Part I as well as in Part II. For reasons of the program's operations, the date entered in Part II, 2.5, must be the same as that in Part I, 2.0.

Preoperative   = period of time from admission to 24.00 hrs on the day before surgery.

Intraoperative = day of surgery.

Perioperative = period of time from the day of surgery to the third day after surgery (included).

Postoperative = period of time from the fourth day after surgery to the day of discharge.

Hb, Hct values: the one available is to be entered; if both available, enter the Hct one; (the transformation from Hb to Hct values will be automatically performed while processing the data); Hb values to be given as g/dL; Hct as a percentage.

The item 'stated reason for transfusion available in patient record' is to be entered with a N/Y answer only if the patient was transfused in the perioperative period, otherwise ignore the field.

The item 'complication of homologous blood transfusion' is to be entered with a N/Y answer only if the patient was transfused with homologous blood units.

The item 'complication of autotransfusion at the donation' is to be entered with a N/Y answer only if the patient donated autologous blood, predeposit and/or haemodilution, otherwise ignore the field.

The item 'complication of autologous blood at the transfusion' is to be entered with a N/Y answer only if the patient was transfused with autologous blood (or if the patient received homologous blood when autologous blood was available), otherwise ignore the field.

4. DEFINITION OF SOME ITEMS (non-ambiguous)

Protocol Part I, II

4.0. Drugs: protocol third and fourth version indicates this item more clearly. Nevertheless, according to the decision taken during the third workshop, the national coordinators will give the 'non-medical data collectors' a list of the 'nonsteroid anti-inflammatory drugs'.

6.0. Anaesthesia: combined, when more than one technique is used.

8.0. Autologous blood procured; refers to units which are available at/during surgery.

10.4. Artificial colloids: HES = Hydroxyethyl starch.

11.0. Stated reason for transfusion available in patient record: reasons upon which the clinicians decided to transfuse in the perioperative period. To complete this table, mark with Y all the items selected, except for anaemia, where the Hct value should be entered.

European Commission

EUR 15398 — Safe and Good Use of Blood in Surgery (SANGUIS) — Use of blood products and artificial colloids in 43 European hospitals

G. Sirchia, A. M. Giovanetti, D. B. L. McClelland, G. N. Fracchia

Luxembourg: Office for Official Publications of the European Communities

1994 — XIV, 235 pp., 49 tab., 167 fig. — 17.6 × 25.0 cm

Medicine and health series

ISBN 92-826-4118-X

Price (excluding VAT) in Luxembourg: ECU 26.50

Venta y suscripciones • Salg og abonnement • Verkauf und Abonnement • Πωλήσεις και συνδρομές
Sales and subscriptions • Vente et abonnements • Vendita e abbonamenti
Verkoop en abonnementen • Venda e assinaturas

BELGIQUE / BELGIË

Moniteur belge /
Belgisch staatsblad
Rue de Louvain 42 / Leuvenseweg 42
1000 Bruxelles / 1000 Brussel
Tél. (02) 512 00 26
Fax (02) 511 01 84

Jean De Lannoy
Avenue du Roi 202 / Koningslaan 202
1060 Bruxelles / 1060 Brussel
Tél. (02) 538 51 69
Télex 63220 UNBOOK B
Fax (02) 538 08 41

Autres distributeurs/
Overige verkooppunten:

Librairie européenne/
Europese boekhandel
Rue de la Loi 244/Wetstraat 244
1040 Bruxelles / 1040 Brussel
Tél. (02) 231 04 35
Fax (02) 735 08 60

Document delivery:

Credoc
Rue de la Montagne 34 / Bergstraat 34
Bte 11 / Bus 11
1000 Bruxelles / 1000 Brussel
Tél. (02) 511 69 41
Fax (02) 513 31 95

DANMARK

J. H. Schultz Information A/S
Herstedvang 10-12
2620 Albertslund
Tlf. 43 63 23 00
Fax (Sales) 43 63 19 69
Fax (Management) 43 63 19 49

DEUTSCHLAND

Bundesanzeiger Verlag
Breite Straße 78-80
Postfach 10 05 34
50445 Köln
Tel. (02 21) 20 29-0
Telex ANZEIGER BONN 8 882 595
Fax 202 92 78

GREECE/ΕΛΛΑΔΑ

G.C. Eleftheroudakis SA
International Bookstore
Nikis Street 4
10563 Athens
Tel. (01) 322 63 23
Telex 219410 ELEF
Fax 323 98 21

ESPAÑA

Boletín Oficial del Estado
Trafalgar, 27-29
28071 Madrid
Tel. (91) 538 22 95
Fax (91) 538 23 49

Mundi-Prensa Libros, SA
Castelló, 37
28001 Madrid
Tel. (91) 431 33 99 (Libros)
431 32 22 (Suscripciones)
435 36 37 (Dirección)
Télex 49370-MPLI-E
Fax (91) 575 39 98

Sucursal:

Librería Internacional AEDOS
Consejo de Ciento, 391
08009 Barcelona
Tel. (93) 488 34 92
Fax (93) 487 76 59

Llibreria de la Generalitat
de Catalunya
Rambla dels Estudis, 118 (Palau Moja)
08002 Barcelona
Tel. (93) 302 68 35
Tel. (93) 302 64 62
Fax (93) 302 12 99

FRANCE

Journal officiel
Service des publications
des Communautés européennes
26, rue Desaix
75727 Paris Cedex 15
Tél. (1) 40 58 77 01/31
Fax (1) 40 58 77 00

IRELAND

Government Supplies Agency
4-5 Harcourt Road
Dublin 2
Tel. (1) 66 13 111
Fax (1) 47 80 645

ITALIA

Licosa SpA
Via Duca di Calabria 1/1
Casella postale 552
50125 Firenze
Tel. (055) 64 54 15
Fax 64 12 57
Telex 570466 LICOSA I

GRAND-DUCHÉ DE LUXEMBOURG

Messageries du livre
5, rue Raiffeisen
2411 Luxembourg
Tél. 40 10 20
Fax 49 06 61

NEDERLAND

SDU Overheidsinformatie
Externe Fondsen
Postbus 20014
2500 EA 's-Gravenhage
Tel. (070) 37 89 880
Fax (070) 37 89 783

PORTUGAL

Imprensa Nacional
Casa da Moeda, EP
Rua D. Francisco Manuel de Melo, 5
1092 Lisboa Codex
Tel. (01) 69 34 14
Fax (01) 69 31 66

Distribuidora de Livros
Bertrand, Ld.ª

Grupo Bertrand, SA
Rua das Terras dos Vales, 4-A
Apartado 37
2700 Amadora Codex
Tel. (01) 49 59 050
Telex 15798 BERDIS
Fax 49 60 255

UNITED KINGDOM

HMSO Books (Agency section)
HMSO Publications Centre
51 Nine Elms Lane
London SW8 5DR
Tel. (071) 873 9090
Fax 873 8463
Telex 29 71 138

ÖSTERREICH

Manz'sche Verlags-
und Universitätsbuchhandlung
Kohlmarkt 16
1014 Wien
Tel. (1) 531 610
Telex 112 500 BOX A
Fax (1) 531 61-181

SUOMI/FINLAND

Akateeminen Kirjakauppa
Keskuskatu 1
PO Box 218
00381 Helsinki
Tel. (0) 121 41
Fax (0) 121 44 41

NORGE

Narvesen Info Center
Bertrand Narvesens vei 2
PO Box 6125 Etterstad
0602 Oslo 6
Tel. (22) 57 33 00
Telex 79668 NIC N
Fax (22) 68 19 01

SVERIGE

BTJ AB
Traktorvgen 13
22100 Lund
Tel. (046) 18 00 00
Fax (046) 18 01 25
30 79 47

ICELAND

BOKABUD
LARUSAR BLÖNDAL
Skólavördustíg, 2
101 Reykjavik
Tel. 11 56 50
Fax 12 55 60

SCHWEIZ / SUISSE / SVIZZERA

OSEC
Stampfenbachstraße 85
8035 Zürich
Tel. (01) 365 54 49
Fax (01) 365 54 11

BÂLGARIJA

Europress Klassica BK
Ltd
66, bd Vitosha
1463 Sofia
Tel./Fax 2 52 74 75

ČESKÁ REPUBLIKA

NIS ČR
Havelkova 22
130 00 Praha 3
Tel. (2) 24 22 94 33
Fax (2) 24 22 14 84

MAGYARORSZÁG

Euro-Info-Service
Honvéd Europá Ház
Margitsziget
1138 Budapest
Tel./Fax 1 111 60 61
1 111 62 16

POLSKA

Business Foundation
ul. Krucza 38/42
00-512 Warszawa
Tel. (2) 621 99 93, 628-28-82
International Fax&Phone
(0-39) 12-00-77

ROMÂNIA

Euromedia
65, Strada Dionisie Lupu
70184 Bucuresti
Tel./Fax 0 12 96 46

RUSSIA

CCEC
9,60-letiya Oktyabrya Avenue
117312 Moscow
Tel./Fax (095) 135 52 27

SLOVAKIA

Slovak Technical
Library
Nm. slobody 19
812 23 Bratislava 1
Tel. (7) 220 452
Fax : (7) 295 785

CYPRUS

Cyprus Chamber of Commerce and
Industry
Chamber Building
38 Grivas Dhigenis Ave
3 Deligiorgis Street
PO Box 1455
Nicosia
Tel. (2) 449500/462312
Fax (2) 458630

MALTA

Miller distributors Ltd
PO Box 25
Malta International Airport
LQA 05 Malta
Tel. 66 44 88
Fax 67 67 99

TÜRKIYE

Pres Gazete Kitap Dergi
Pazarlama Dagitim Ticaret ve sanayi
AŞ
Narlibaçhe Sokak N. 15
Istanbul-Cagaloğlu
Tel. (1) 520 92 96 - 528 55 66
Fax 520 64 57
Telex 23822 DSVO-TR

ISRAEL

ROY International
PO Box 13056
41 Mishmar Hayarden Street
Tel Aviv 61130
Tel. 3 496 108
Fax 3 648 60 39

EGYPT/
MIDDLE EAST

Middle East Observer
41 Sherif St.
Cairo
Tel/Fax 39 39 732

UNITED STATES OF AMERICA /
CANADA

UNIPUB
4611-F Assembly Drive
Lanham, MD 20706-4391
Tel. Toll Free (800) 274 4888
Fax (301) 459 0056

CANADA

Subscriptions only
Uniquement abonnements

Renouf Publishing Co. Ltd
1294 Algoma Road
Ottawa, Ontario K1B 3W8
Tel. (613) 741 43 33
Fax (613) 741 54 39
Telex 0534783

AUSTRALIA

Hunter Publications
58A Gipps Street
Collingwood
Victoria 3066
Tel. (3) 417 5361
Fax (3) 419 7154

JAPAN

Kinokuniya Company Ltd
17-7 Shinjuku 3-Chome
Shinjuku-ku
Tokyo 160-91
Tel. (03) 3439-0121

Journal Department
PO Box 55 Chitose
Tokyo 156
Tel. (03) 3439-0124

SOUTH-EAST ASIA

Legal Library Services Ltd
Orchard
PO Box 0523
Singapore 9123
Tel. 73 04 24 1
Fax 24 32 47 9

SOUTH AFRICA

Safto
5th Floor, Export House
Cnr Maude & West Streets
Sandton 2146
Tel. (011) 883-3737
Fax (011) 883-6569

AUTRES PAYS
OTHER COUNTRIES
ANDERE LÄNDER

Office des publications officielles
des Communautés européennes
2, rue Mercier
2985 Luxembourg
Tél. 499 28-1
Télex PUBOF LU 1324 b
Fax 48 85 73/48 68 17

6/94